Overcoming Common Problems

Eating for a Healthy Heart

Robert Povey, Jacqui Morrell and Rachel Povey

sheldon **PRESS**

First published in Great Britain in 2005

Sheldon Press
36 Causton Street
London SW1P 4ST

Copyright © Robert Povey, Jacqui Morrell and Rachel Povey 2005
Illustrations copyright © Marilyn Rix 2005

The authors and publisher have made every effort to ensure that
the external website addresses included in this book are correct
and up to date at the time of going to press. The authors and
publisher are not responsible for the content, quality or
continuing accessibility of the sites.

British Library Cataloguing-in-Publication Data

A catalogue record for this book is available from the British Library

ISBN 0–85969–895–5

1 3 5 7 9 10 8 6 4 2

Typeset by Deltatype Limited, Birkenhead, Merseyside
Printed in Great Britain by Ashford Colour Press

DR ROBERT POVEY is a freelance psychologist and author of *How to Keep Your Cholesterol in Check* (Sheldon Press, 2005, 3rd edition), the companion book to *Eating for a Healthy Heart*. Formerly Principal Lecturer in Psychology at Christ Church College, Canterbury, and a qualified nurse, he has written several books and articles on topics in psychology and health. Having had to cope personally with the need to modify cholesterol levels by diet, he has gained valuable first-hand experience of ways in which to prepare healthy meals that can help in the prevention of heart disease.

JACQUI MORRELL is a State Registered Dietitian with a BSc in Dietetics. She works at the Conquest Hospital, Hastings, and has a specialist interest in the prevention and treatment of heart disease. She was also, for many years, dietitian at H·E·A·R·T UK, formerly the Family Heart Association. She has written several articles and scientific papers on how to cope with dietary problems in heart disease and, as Jacqui Lynas, she wrote two cookbooks – *The Heart of Delicious Cooking* (Pulse Medical Publishing/Guy's and St Thomas' Hospital Trust, 1994) and *Cooking for a Healthy Heart* (Hamlyn, 2002). She also co-authored, with Paul Gayler, *Healthy Eating for Your Heart* (Kyle Cathie, 2003).

DR RACHEL POVEY is a Chartered Health Psychologist and Senior Lecturer in Health Psychology at Staffordshire University. She has undertaken extensive research into the problems people experience in attempting to adopt and maintain healthy diets. She has worked with both healthy individuals and people needing to keep to strict dietary regimes. Her early work at the University of Leeds formed part of the research programme resulting in the report *The Nation's Diet* and her work on dietary factors in diabetes has been carried out under the auspices of the European Association for the Study of Diabetes.

Overcoming Common Problems Series

Selected titles
A full list of titles is available from Sheldon Press,
36 Causton Street, London SW1P 4ST, and on our website at
www.sheldonpress.co.uk

Assertiveness: Step by Step
Dr Windy Dryden and Daniel Constantinou

Body Language at Work
Mary Hartley

The Cancer Guide for Men
Helen Beare and Neil Priddy

The Candida Diet Book
Karen Brody

The Chronic Fatigue Healing Diet
Christine Craggs-Hinton

Cider Vinegar
Margaret Hills

Comfort for Depression
Janet Horwood

Confidence Works
Gladeana McMahon

Coping Successfully with Hay Fever
Dr Robert Youngson

Coping Successfully with Pain
Neville Shone

Coping Successfully with Panic Attacks
Shirley Trickett

Coping Successfully with Prostate Cancer
Dr Tom Smith

Coping Successfully with Prostate Problems
Rosy Reynolds

Coping Successfully with RSI
Maggie Black and Penny Gray

Coping Successfully with Your Hiatus Hernia
Dr Tom Smith

Coping with Alopecia
Dr Nigel Hunt and Dr Sue McHale

Coping with Anxiety and Depression
Shirley Trickett

Coping with Blushing
Dr Robert Edelmann

Coping with Bronchitis and Emphysema
Dr Tom Smith

Coping with Candida
Shirley Trickett

Coping with Childhood Asthma
Jill Eckersley

Coping with Chronic Fatigue
Trudie Chalder

Coping with Coeliac Disease
Karen Brody

Coping with Cystitis
Caroline Clayton

Coping with Depression and Elation
Dr Patrick McKeon

Coping with Down's Syndrome
Fiona Marshall

Coping with Dyspraxia
Jill Eckersley

Coping with Eczema
Dr Robert Youngson

Coping with Endometriosis
Jo Mears

Coping with Epilepsy
Fiona Marshall and
Dr Pamela Crawford

Coping with Fibroids
Mary-Claire Mason

Coping with Gallstones
Dr Joan Gomez

Coping with Gout
Christine Craggs-Hinton

Coping with a Hernia
Dr David Delvin

Coping with Incontinence
Dr Joan Gomez

Coping with Long-Term Illness
Barbara Baker

Coping with the Menopause
Janet Horwood

Coping with a Mid-life Crisis
Derek Milne

Coping with Polycystic Ovary Syndrome
Christine Craggs-Hinton

Coping with Psoriasis
Professor Ronald Marks

Overcoming Common Problems Series

Coping with SAD
Fiona Marshall and Peter Cheevers

Coping with Snoring and Sleep Apnoea
Jill Eckersley

Coping with Stomach Ulcers
Dr Tom Smith

Coping with Strokes
Dr Tom Smith

Coping with Suicide
Maggie Helen

Coping with Teenagers
Sarah Lawson

Coping with Thyroid Problems
Dr Joan Gomez

Curing Arthritis – The Drug-Free Way
Margaret Hills

Curing Arthritis – More Ways to a Drug-Free Life
Margaret Hills

Curing Arthritis Diet Book
Margaret Hills

Curing Arthritis Exercise Book
Margaret Hills and Janet Horwood

Cystic Fibrosis – A Family Affair
Jane Chumbley

Depression at Work
Vicky Maud

Depressive Illness
Dr Tim Cantopher

Effortless Exercise
Dr Caroline Shreeve

Fertility
Julie Reid

The Fibromyalgia Healing Diet
Christine Craggs-Hinton

Getting a Good Night's Sleep
Fiona Johnston

The Good Stress Guide
Mary Hartley

Heal the Hurt: How to Forgive and Move On
Dr Ann Macaskill

Heart Attacks – Prevent and Survive
Dr Tom Smith

Helping Children Cope with Attention Deficit Disorder
Dr Patricia Gilbert

Helping Children Cope with Bullying
Sarah Lawson

Helping Children Cope with Change and Loss
Rosemary Wells

Helping Children Cope with Divorce
Rosemary Wells

Helping Children Cope with Grief
Rosemary Wells

Helping Children Cope with Stammering
Jackie Turnbull and Trudy Stewart

Helping Children Get the Most from School
Sarah Lawson

How to Accept Yourself
Dr Windy Dryden

How to Be Your Own Best Friend
Dr Paul Hauck

How to Cope with Anaemia
Dr Joan Gomez

How to Cope with Bulimia
Dr Joan Gomez

How to Cope with Stress
Dr Peter Tyrer

How to Enjoy Your Retirement
Vicky Maud

How to Improve Your Confidence
Dr Kenneth Hambly

How to Keep Your Cholesterol in Check
Dr Robert Povey

How to Lose Weight Without Dieting
Mark Barker

How to Make Yourself Miserable
Dr Windy Dryden

How to Pass Your Driving Test
Donald Ridland

How to Stand up for Yourself
Dr Paul Hauck

How to Stick to a Diet
Deborah Steinberg and Dr Windy Dryden

How to Stop Worrying
Dr Frank Tallis

The How to Study Book
Alan Brown

How to Succeed as a Single Parent
Carole Baldock

How to Untangle Your Emotional Knots
Dr Windy Dryden and Jack Gordon

Hysterectomy
Suzie Hayman

Overcoming Common Problems Series

Contents

Acknowledgements

We would like to say a special thank you to our other halves – Lyn, Jonathan and Andy – for their constant support and encouragement during the writing of the book, and to Lottie, Sam and Tom for testing recipes and giving us the teenager's point of view. We are also grateful to Liz Marsh, formerly Commissioning Editor at Sheldon Press, for the enthusiastic backing she gave to the book, from preliminary discussions right through to the final draft; and to H·E·A·R·T UK and its Director, Michael Livingston, for their keen interest and involvement in the project and for agreeing to endorse the book.

Most of the quotes in the book have been adapted from survey interviews conducted by Dr Rachel Povey in collaboration with Dr Mark Conner, Dr Paul Sparks, Dr Richard Shepherd and Ms Rhiannon James, as part of the project 'Ambivalence about health-related dietary change'. This was funded by the Economic and Social Research Council in the UK as part of *The Nation's Diet* programme. The quotes have been modified where necessary to preserve the participants' anonymity.

We are also grateful to the British Heart Foundation and the Stroke Association for permission to reproduce or adapt text from some of their publications.

A proportion of the royalties from the book are being donated to support the work of H·E·A·R·T UK.

Introduction

'Not another book telling us we can't eat this and we can't eat that!' This is a reaction we often come across, and it's true that some people do react strongly against any idea of 'healthy eating' because they imagine that this will involve having to give up all the gastronomic delights they currently enjoy. Fortunately, this is very rarely the case. Although some people may need to introduce a few modifications to their current eating habits for medical reasons, these can usually be handled in such a way that, rather than being penalties, they become opportunities to try new, exciting foods and drinks that will taste good as well as provide extra benefits for our health.

This book is designed as a companion volume to *How to Keep Your Cholesterol in Check* by Dr Robert Povey (Sheldon Press, 2005, 3rd edition), which deals in detail with the principles and practice behind the development of a healthy, cholesterol-lowering lifestyle, including diet. In this book, therefore, we have only examined the most important details about the relationship between diet and heart health, concentrating on the practical aspects of eating a healthy diet and leaving those of our readers who wish to pursue the issue in greater depth to refer to the companion volume.

The initial chapters look at the ways in which our bodies deal with different types of food and drink – from fats and fibre, to alcohol and antioxidants. Here we also offer advice on how to choose the best types of food and drink to protect our hearts, keep a healthy weight for a healthy heart, change dietary habits where necessary and make such changes more manageable. We hope that the book will be helpful to those people who simply wish to eat more healthily as well as those who have to deal with medical conditions affecting the functioning of the heart.

The second part of the book offers a range of healthy recipes that you can incorporate into your own repertoire of creative cooking. There are no single right answers in cookery – it's a matter of experimenting with basic recipes until you find the blend of ingredients and style of cooking that suits you best. We hope that the book will help in this process and that you enjoy the results.

1
How food and drink affect the heart

The heart is our engine room, constantly driving blood around the body to enable it to function smoothly and effectively. Fresh blood, oxygenated by the lungs, is pumped through the arteries, nourishing the body's organs with oxygen. We are able to determine, to some extent at least, how this crucial pump is maintained and, thus, we can exercise some control over the health of our bodies. The type and quantity of food and drink we ingest can be regarded as forming the basic constituents of the 'fuel' we decide to use to 'stoke up' the engine. If we use the right sort of fuel, backed up by a healthy lifestyle, we can help the engine to operate smoothly and efficiently. As one of the interviewees in *The Nation's Diet* research programme put it, 'I think it would be better for your heart and things like that, you know, to be a healthy eater. I should imagine you'd be fitter.' If we use the wrong type of fuel, though – especially in large quantities – then this can interfere with the proper functioning of our engine room, clogging up the arteries and making the heart's life-sustaining role much more difficult to maintain.

Cholesterol

One of the most common ways in which the choice of inappropriate 'fuel' can affect the heart and its related blood vessels (the *cardiovascular system*) is through the build-up of *cholesterol* deposits in the arteries. Too much of the wrong types of fuel, usually in the form of saturated fats, causes the arteries to narrow over a period of time. This results in a rise in blood pressure, so the heart finds greater and greater difficulty in pumping blood around the body. Then people often start to experience pain in the chest on exertion (*angina*). This is the heart muscle's way of telling us that it is finding it difficult to work properly because it is being starved of oxygen.

The tendency for people to develop heart problems is not entirely related to our eating habits or lifestyles, of course. It's determined by a combination of factors, including the characteristics that we inherit as well as the lifestyles we lead. In some cases, people are born with an inherited genetic disorder in which levels of cholesterol in the blood are excessively raised. This disorder – called *familial hypercholesterolaemia* or *FH* – affects about 1 in 500 people and requires careful management. However, even problems like this can be handled effectively with a combination of drugs and dietary modifications. People with FH have to make sure that they keep their intake of saturated fat to within their individually recommended limits, but, in general, they will find that the recipes included in this book provide an excellent basis for their own low-fat culinary explorations.

Further details about cholesterol problems and how to deal with them can be found in the companion volume *How to Keep Your Cholesterol in Check*. For people wishing to receive personal advice about FH and/or regular updates on current developments in the treatment of heart disease, the association H·E·A·R·T UK exists for just this purpose. Its staff will be delighted to welcome you on board. You don't have to suffer from FH to become a member. If you're interested in finding out about ways in which to prevent heart disease and would like to support a lively and worthwhile charity, H·E·A·R·T UK can be contacted on 01628 628638, e-mailed at <info@heartuk.org.uk> or you can visit the website at <www.heartuk.org>.

The role of cholesterol in our bodies

Cholesterol is frequently seen as something that has entirely harmful effects whereas, in reality, it forms an essential component of the membranes of all the cells in our bodies. In fact, we cannot live without it. This white waxy substance is used to make bile, which plays an important role in the digestion of fatty foods. It also helps to produce various hormones and vitamin D, and to insulate our nerves. About two-thirds of our cholesterol is made in the liver, using substances derived from the fat in our food. So, the more fat we eat, the more cholesterol is produced. The type of fat that most strongly encourages the production of cholesterol is *saturated* fat, found for the most part in foods derived from animal sources, such as full-cream milk, butter, lard and fatty meat or cheese. A small proportion of the body's cholesterol is called *dietary cholesterol* because it is contained in, and comes directly from, the food we eat, such as meat and egg yolks. Its role is relatively insignificant in the development of cholesterol-related health problems, although people with severe problems are usually advised to restrict their intake of egg yolks to two a week. However, most cholesterol problems arise because of

2

too high an intake of *saturated* fat and we shall offer some advice on choosing various types of fat in the next chapter.

Different forms of cholesterol

Cholesterol reaches the body's cells via the bloodstream, carried in tiny packages called *lipoproteins*. We don't need to go into too much detail about these, except to say that lipoproteins differ in density – one type of cholesterol is *low-density lipoprotein* (LDL) and another *high-density lipoprotein* (HDL). It is helpful to become familiar with these because, as someone put it in a *Family Heart Association* newsletter (now the *H·E·A·R·T UK Digest*), one type is a *Less Desirable Lipoprotein* (LDL) and the other a *Highly Desirable Lipoprotein* (HDL).

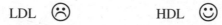

LDL ☹   HDL ☺

People who have a lot of LDL cholesterol in their blood have a high risk of building up deposits that fur up their arteries and increase the risk of heart disease. Having a good supply of HDL cholesterol, however, actually protects you from heart disease. It seems that HDL cholesterol acts a bit like a scavenger, collecting up surplus cholesterol from the arteries and taking it back to the liver where it can be reprocessed as bile. We shall return to these different types of cholesterol in the next chapter, when we will find that we can increase the highly desirable HDL cholesterol at the expense of the less desirable LDL by taking care when deciding on the kinds of cooking ingredients we use (especially the fats), what we choose to drink, and the frequency and type of exercise we take.

Before we leave lipoproteins (lipids for short), we need just to mention one more type – these are the very low-density lipids that mainly contain *triglycerides*. These again are either made in the liver or come from fat in foods. They form an important source of fuel for our bodies, but, in excess, can lead to an increased tendency to suffer from blood clots and coronary heart disease. The level of triglycerides in the blood can also be controlled to some extent by our choice of food and drink, and people with raised triglyceride levels (often related to diabetes or obesity) need to keep intakes of alcohol and sugar low and increase the types of foods that have the effect of decreasing their triglycerides, such as oily fish or fish oil supplements.

As a rough rule of thumb you should aim to keep your:

- total cholesterol level down to below 5.0 mmol/L (195 mg/dL)
- LDL below 3.0 mmol/L (115 mg/dL)
- HDL above 1.0 mmol/L (40 mg/dL)
- triglyceride levels below 1.5 mmol/L (57mg/dL).

These measurements (obtained from a blood test) are explained in detail in *How to Keep Your Cholesterol in Check*. The guidelines are revised from time to time (and are slightly more stringent compared with those used in earlier editions of the companion book). They represent the current recommendations set out by national guidelines and the opinions of medical experts in the field.

The next chapter looks at how our choice of fats and fibres can help in improving our lipid profiles.

2
Carbohydrates, fibre and fats

The types and amounts of fat and fibre we eat have a big effect on how well our bodies work and the shapes they turn into! If you turn into an apple shape, with your fat deposited around the stomach like a pot belly, you are more at risk of heart disease than if you are pear-shaped, with your fat distributed over your hips and thighs. When fat cells concentrate around the stomach, they make the body more resistant to the hormone insulin. So, in order to compensate for this, we produce more insulin and this tends to be associated with increases in blood pressure, triglycerides and total cholesterol. There is also an increased likelihood of blood clotting and, of course, developing diabetes.

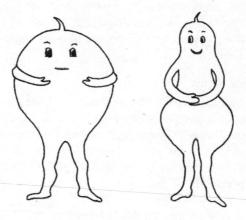

You can calculate whether you are apple- or pear-shaped (if you can't see it by looking in the mirror!) by dividing your waist measurement by your hip measurement. A high ratio puts you in the apple group and a low ratio in the pear-shaped group. If your waist to hip ratio is more than 1.0 for men or 0.8 for women, this puts you at increased risk of developing cardiovascular disease and diabetes. This means, generally, that you should aim to keep your waist size below your hip size. For men, the same size waist and hip just keeps them within their advised ratio of 1.0, but, for women, waist size needs to be several centimetres smaller than the size of their naturally broader hips in order to keep to a ratio of 0.8 or below. So, for example, a woman with a 112-cm (44-inch) hip measurement would need to aim for a waist measurement of 89 cm (35 inches) or below (89 ÷ 112 = 0.8).

Carbohydrates

To keep the waist–hip ratio to a reasonable figure, it is very helpful to know more about the effects different foods have on our bodies and the effects of different carbohydrates are especially relevant here. *Simple carbohydrates* (sugars) are found in sweet foods, such as cakes and pastries, and provide lots of energy-producing calories that can be burnt off provided we take enough exercise. On the other hand, the so-called *complex carbohydrates* (starches), found in foods of plant origin, such as cereals, pulses, fruits and vegetables, also provide energy, but release it more slowly as they take a long time to be digested and absorbed into the body. These are generally helpful for keeping our hearts in good shape, our bowels in good working order and our weight in check. They are also an important source of vitamins and minerals.

The glycaemic index

There is a select group of foods within the category of complex carbohydrates that have been shown to have particularly beneficial effects on our bodies. These are known as foods with a low *glycaemic index* (GI). They help to decrease the risk of diabetes by controlling both our weight and blood glucose levels and they protect our arteries from furring up by increasing the level of good HDL cholesterol in the blood.

Foods with a low GI index are favoured by athletes because they provide the benefit of a slow and sustained release of glucose that occurs even during exercise. This enables the athlete to exercise for much longer before fatigue sets in than is possible after having eaten other foods. (A useful website from which you can obtain details about the GI of individual foods and an indication of whether these are low, medium or high can be found at <www.glycemicindex.com>.)

Some good examples of low-fat foods with a low GI are:

- oats and bran
- lentils

- pasta
- basmati rice and couscous
- beans, including baked beans, but soya and kidney beans are especially low
- multi-wholegrain breads made with, for example, barley, rye, linseeds, sunflower seeds, oats, soy, kibbled wheat
- skimmed milk
- low-fat yogurt
- apples, oranges, grapefruit
- apricots, pears, peaches, plums, cherries.

So it's a good idea to base your meals and snacks around complex carbohydrates and look out for foods with a low GI where possible. This is particularly important for people who tend to have raised blood glucose levels, but we can all benefit from keeping the balance of our food intake on the low side as far as the GI index is concerned. So, choose basmati or wholegrain rice, for example, rather than white rice, oat- or bran-based cereals rather than corn-flakes, and pasta or new potatoes rather than baked potatoes. The latter are, surprisingly, higher on the index than new potatoes, sweet potatoes and yams (these are similar to sweet potatoes but slightly more moist), largely because they contain lower amounts of the slowly digested starch amylose. However, baked potatoes (like other foods with a highish GI) are still an excellent source of complex carbohydrates.

The point to remember is that it's the balance of the *whole* meal that is important as far as the GI is concerned. A meal that combines both low and medium-to-high GI foods will still leave you with a balanced, intermediate GI intake. So, don't write off having a baked potato just because it has a highish GI. Your choice of accompanying food, such as Bean goulash or Ratatouille (see the Recipes section) can easily bring down the overall index for the whole meal to an acceptable level. Potatoes in all shapes and sizes, together with wholegrain bread, cereals, rice, pasta and pulses, should certainly be seen as an important element in a nourishing, low-fat, heart-healthy diet. Such complex carbohydrates provide an excellent source of dietary fibre, both soluble and insoluble (see pages 8–9). They also help to ensure a good supply of energy (especially important when you are reducing the fat content of your diet), vitamins and minerals. Pulses, such as soya and kidney beans, also provide us with plenty of protein, which is essential for the growth and repair of body tissues.

Low-carbohydrate diets

There has been a lot of publicity about low-carbohydrate and high-protein diets (the Atkins diet, for example) and it's true that you can sometimes achieve quite dramatic weight loss in this way. Starved of carbohydrates, the body needs to get its energy from other sources, so it burns off its fat stores – a process that happens with most slimming diets. It also appears that a high protein intake may have the effect of reducing overall appetite levels. So, in the short term, these diets might work, assuming that you can put up with the possibility of unpleasant side-effects, such as headaches and bad breath.

The main problems are likely to be in the longer term. For example, these diets tend to encourage only a selected intake of fruit and vegetables – those with a low carbohydrate content. If you continue to follow this eating pattern over a long period, there is a danger that you will starve the body of important vitamins and fibre that are obtained from eating a range of fruit and vegetables and other carbohydrates. The lack of such heart-protective nutrients and the surfeit of saturated fat these diets contain may increase the likelihood of developing cardiovascular problems in the future. Low carbohydrate intake combined with an excess of protein can also result in minerals such as calcium being leached from the bones, making them more fragile. Not enough people have been on the Atkins diet yet for doctors to be able to assess the true long-term health risks, but many members of the dietetic and medical professions do feel unease at the restrictions of this diet. They would argue that, in order to maintain a healthy body and healthy heart, we should stick to a low-fat, well-balanced diet, including carbohydrates, and a lifestyle that involves regular physical activity. This is the approach we recommend in this book.

Fibre – soluble and insoluble

Dietary fibre is key to maintaining a healthy digestion and regular bowel movements, but it also plays an important role in keeping down total cholesterol levels and, hence, reducing problems with the heart.

Some fibre is *insoluble*. This means that it doesn't dissolve, but will absorb water and swell up to give bulk to the stools, helping to prevent constipation. The remainder is *soluble*, but it does not break down sufficiently to be absorbed into the bloodstream. What it does do very effectively, however, is form a sort of sticky gel that slows down the food's passage through the body. By doing this it helps to reduce the release of sugar into the bloodstream and also retains some of the bile acids, preventing them from being reabsorbed. This results in more of the liver-produced cholesterol being used to replace the 'lost' bile and this, in turn, reduces the amount of total cholesterol in the blood.

The different types of fibre and their effects are summarized in Table 2.1.

Table 2.1 Types of fibre and their effects on the body

Type of fibre	Examples of relevant foods	Effect on the body
Soluble	Rolled oats, oat bran, oat-based cereals and breads Peas, split peas, lentils, chickpeas, soya beans and baked beans Some fruits – apples, dates, strawberries and citrus fruits	Lowers total cholesterol
Insoluble	Wholegrain bread and cereals Brown rice Wholewheat pasta Fruit and vegetables with edible skins and seeds	Prevents bowel problems

Fats

There are three main types of fat in food – *saturates*, *polyunsaturates* and *monounsaturates*. All the fats we come across in food are a mixture of these three basic types, sometimes together with *trans-fatty acids* (also called *trans-fats*). These trans-fats are produced as a result of a process called *hydrogenation* – used to convert unsaturated vegetable oils into solid fat suitable for use in baking or for spreading. They are found in lots of margarines, biscuits and cakes and our bodies react to them in much the same way that they react to saturates.

Fats and oils are essentially similar, both consisting of fatty acids, which are substances used by the body for energy and tissue development. However, fats are solid or semi-solid at room temperature whereas oils are liquid.

They are good sources of energy, but too much fat of the wrong type can be damaging to health and to our hearts. *Saturated* fats – mostly found in foods of animal origin – tend to be the main culprits when it comes to raising our total cholesterol levels. The unsaturated fats tend to help keep our cholesterol levels down, as do the low-fat spreads (or foods) fortified with *plant stanols* or *sterols*.

Essential fatty acids

It's worth noting two of the specific polyunsaturated fatty acids we need to obtain from the foods we eat. They are *linoleic* and *alpha-linolenic acids* and are called *essential fatty acids* because they are the only fatty acids that are essential to health and cannot be manufactured within our bodies.

They belong to the *omega-6* and *omega-3* families of fatty acids, respectively. Both these families of fatty acids have beneficial effects on heart health, but work in different ways. You may have come across them in advertisements for certain foods.

Omega-3 fatty acids are mainly derived from *alpha-linolenic acid* and are found in:

- oily fish
- flax seeds (linseed), rapeseed, soya beans, walnuts and their oils and margarines
- dark green leafy vegetables, such as spinach
- eggs from hens fed on omega-3-rich diets.

These fatty acids can help to prevent potentially fatal heart arrhythmias (abnormal heart rhythms) and thrombosis (blood clots) and they reduce inflammation and triglyceride levels. They may also lower blood pressure and increase the good HDL cholesterol.

Omega-6 fatty acids, on the other hand, are mainly derived from *linoleic acid* and are found in sunflower, safflower, corn, and soya

Table 2.2 The effects of the different fats on heart health

Type of fat	Examples of relevant foods	Effect on heart health
Saturated fats	Fatty meats, whole milk, cream, hard cheese and full-fat soft cheese, butter, lard, hard margarines, suet and palm oil, many prepacked convenience foods; biscuits, cakes, pastries, crisps and take-away foods	☹ Raise total cholesterol
Trans-fats	Mainly found in hydrogenated vegetable oils, some margarines and in commercially prepared foods, such as biscuits; small amounts also in the fat of dairy products and some meats	☹ Raise total cholesterol
Polyunsaturated fats	Vegetable oils, such as sunflower, corn, safflower, soya, grapeseed, nut oils Many margarines and spreads contain omega-6 fatty acids Omega-3 fatty acids are found in rapeseed, flax seed (linseed) and soya oils, oily fish (e.g. herring, mackerel, salmon, sardines, tuna), walnuts, sweet potatoes, pumpkin, splnach and leafy vegetables	☺ Lower total cholesterol ☺ Reduce blood stickiness ☺ Reduce triglycerides Protect heart from arrhythmias
Monounsaturated fats	Olive and rapeseed (canola) oil, peanut oil and spreads, avocados, many nuts	☺ Lower total cholesterol
Plant stanols or sterols	Some margarines and other foods, such as yogurt, milk and spreading cheese, are made with these plant extracts	☺ Lower total cholesterol They have the effect of displacing cholesterol in the gut

bean oils, margarines and related products. This family of fatty acids actually helps to lower cholesterol.

It has been recognized that keeping a good balance between omega-6 and omega-3 fatty acids in the diet is important for health generally, but especially for good heart health. Our ancestors evolved a diet that contained an equal balance of omega-6 and omega-3, but the modern diet has been shown to contain too much omega-6 and not enough omega-3. To adjust the balance, we need to favour foods high in omega-3 fatty acids when choosing ingredients for a heart-healthy diet.

We have summarized in Table 2.2 (on page 11) the main effects of the different fats in helping to maintain a healthy heart.

In trying to keep a balanced, heart-friendly intake of food, we need to look a little more closely at the sources of *hidden* fats, the high levels of saturated fats that are concealed behind labels such as '80 per cent fat free' and 'low in sugar'. We will look at the problems of hidden fats later on in Chapter 4 on food labelling, but our next task is to explore how we can increase our intake of antioxidants as a way of fighting heart disease.

3
The role of antioxidants

Fruit and vegetables are high in vitamins and minerals and help to fight off infections. These high-fibre foods also provide a rich source of nutrients that can play a role in preventing cholesterol deposits building up in our arteries. Collectively, these nutrients are called *antioxidants* and there are about 600 of them in total. They include some vitamins, in particular beta-carotene (a form of vitamin A), vitamin C and vitamin E – the ACE trio – and minerals selenium and zinc.

Other compounds – flavonoids and phenols, which give fruit and vegetables their colour – are also potent antioxidants. They are present in wine (especially red wine), grape juice and tea. Other good sources of flavonoids are citrus fruits, grapes, cherries, broccoli, tomatoes and onions. Tomatoes and tomato sauce are also rich in lycopene, a nutrient from the same family as beta-carotene, and it has been shown to have excellent antioxidant properties.

When fat goes rancid, this is caused by *oxidization*. The same thing can happen to substances in the body, like cholesterol. When this happens, the cholesterol becomes much more likely to adhere to the artery walls, so antioxidants are an important defence against *atherosclerosis* – the process by which the artery walls become narrowed. They also help to mop up dangerous *free radicals* – the chemical agents that encourage the process of oxidization and are implicated in a number of diseases, including cancer.

Research shows that people who have high intakes of foods with antioxidant properties (see Table 3.1 (on page 14)) tend to have a lower risk of heart disease and cancer than people whose diets are low in these foods.

Eat a rainbow

You can get some idea of the nutritional benefits of different types of fruits and vegetables by looking at their colour and the Stroke Association encourages us to 'Eat a rainbow, beat a stroke'. Eating fruits and vegetables reflecting the colours of a rainbow gives us excellent protection from heart disease and stroke.

Table 3.1 Where to find key antioxidants

Antioxidants	Examples of foods containing them
Beta-carotene (a form of vitamin A)	Carrots, dark green leafy vegetables (such as spinach), apricots, mangoes, melons, red peppers, broccoli, watercress, lettuce It is not destroyed by cooking
Vitamin C (ascorbic acid)	Widely available in fresh fruit and vegetables, but especially good sources are citrus fruits, blackcurrants, strawberries, guavas, broccoli, greens, parsley, peppers and new potatoes Partly destroyed by cooking or exposure to air
Vitamin E	Vegetable oils, especially sunflower seed oil, and margarines, wholemeal cereals, dark green leafy vegetables, such as broccoli and spinach, oily fish, eggs and nuts It is not destroyed by cooking
Selenium	Cereals, fish and nuts, especially Brazil and walnuts It is not destroyed by cooking

- **Red** tomatoes and watermelons contain lycopene.
- **Orange** mangoes and oranges contain plenty of vitamin C and carrots and sweet potatoes are rich in beta-carotene.
- **Yellow** sweetcorn, pineapples and yellow peppers contain the antioxidant lutein, which keeps free radicals at bay and also helps to keep our eyes healthy. Bananas provide potassium, which prevents heart irregularities.
- **Green** broccoli, cabbage, Brussels sprouts and watercress contain folic acid and this helps to keep down the blood levels of

homocysteine, too much of which can lead to damage to the walls of the arteries.

- **Blue** blueberries, blackberries and prunes contain anthocyanin, which may have a role to play in improving circulation. These fruits are also full of heart-healthy vitamins.
- **Indigo or violet** beetroot, aubergines, plums and red cabbage contain a deep red pigment that has powerful antioxidant effects.

The Mediterranean diet

People who live in Mediterranean areas, such as the south of France, southern Italy and Greece, tend to have some of the lowest rates of coronary heart disease in Europe. It seems likely that their diet is one of the main factors contributing to this good heart health.

The Mediterranean diet is especially high in antioxidants, obtained from the rich variety of fruit and vegetables used. Also, a glass or two of red wine with meals is favoured and most of the cooking involves olive oil, which consists mainly of monounsaturates that tend to lower total and less desirable LDL cholesterol levels without decreasing the highly desirable HDL. So, it makes good sense that a Mediterranean-style diet is associated with healthy hearts.

The only paradox – sometimes called the French paradox – is that French people also tend to eat a lot of saturated fat – contained, for example, in soft cheeses – and yet they still have a low incidence of coronary heart disease. The most likely explanation for this apparent anomaly is that the high fat intake is counterbalanced by their even higher consumption of fresh fruit and vegetables, a tendency to drink wine with meals, and the fact that soft cheeses are also high in folic acid, which helps to reduce our risk levels for coronary heart disease. Also, because of their higher water content, soft French cheeses are often lower in fat than hard cheeses. So Camembert, for example, contains 24 per cent fat compared with 33 per cent in Cheddar. However, you need to check the labels for individual varieties.

So, there are some very sound reasons for following a Mediterranean-style diet. Here are some of the recommended elements.

- Eat a variety of complex carbohydrates, for example bread – especially wholemeal and granary – cereals, potatoes, pasta, rice.
- Plenty of fresh fruit and vegetables, eaten raw or lightly cooked.
- Lots of fresh salads.

- Cook with oil high in monounsaturates, such as olive oil.
- Steam, bake or grill rather than deep-fat fry food.
- White and oily fish and small quantities of lean cuts of meat.
- Use garlic (a cholesterol-lowering agent) as an important cooking ingredient.
- Plenty of herbs and spices, but remember to keep quantities of salt low as it raises blood pressure.
- Drink wine (especially red) in moderation with meals.
- Eat at leisure, rather than wolf down fast food snacks while on the move.
- Enjoy and savour the aroma, flavour and taste of foods that are contributing to good heart health.

Five portions of fruit and vegetables a day

One way to ensure that you're getting your daily intake of antioxidants is to follow the advice to eat at least five portions of fruit and vegetables a day. As well as having antioxidant properties, fruit and vegetables are good sources of potassium – a mineral that may help to control blood pressure and prevent irregular heart rhythms. They are also rich in folic acid, which helps to reduce the blood level of a substance called homocysteine and this, as mentioned earlier, is another risk factor in heart disease.

Five portions add up to about 500 g (just over 1 lb) in weight and one portion looks something like the size of a clenched fist. They can include frozen, dried and tinned as well as fresh fruit and vegetables. Note, however, that potatoes are not included as vegetables when following the five portions advice – they count as starchy foods.

Here are some examples of what a portion looks like:

- one large fruit, such as an apple, orange or banana
- two small fruits, such as a couple of plums or clementines
- a medium-sized mug of raspberries, strawberries or grapes
- half to one tablespoon of dried fruit
- two tablespoons of raw, cooked or frozen vegetables
- one cereal bowlful of salad
- one small glass of fruit juice, but only one glass of fruit juice counts as a portion of fruit each day.

We should aim to eat fresh foods whenever possible because the nutritional content is likely to be the most beneficial. We also know exactly what we are eating. We all buy food from the supermarket as well, though, and it's important that we read the labels of foods to check the exact nature of the ingredients because the advertising can be grossly misleading. This is why, next, we look at checking food labels.

4
Checking food labels

To the average shopper, food labels can be something of a minefield. Adverts for different foodstuffs are often skilfully written so that they appear to be offering healthy foods when they are anything but. Don't be fooled, '80 per cent fat free' is still 20 per cent fat. Similarly, '50 per cent reduced fat' may remain a very high total fat, depending on the amount there was to start with. For example, 50 per cent reduced fat (that is, half) of a 60 per cent starting point still leaves 30 per cent fat. Something can legitimately be 'low fat' but still be 'high sugar' or 'high salt'. So, when we're shopping for a healthy heart, we need to be canny food detectives, checking the labels to find out the facts behind the hype. In order to know how much fat or sugar or salt we are eating, we need to know a bit about the nutritional details of the foods we buy.

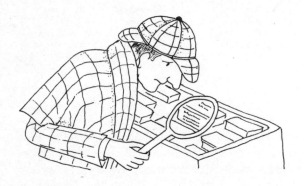

How information is presented

Processed foods have to have an *ingredients* label listing the basic contents and these are given in order of weight. So, the main ingredient is shown first on the list and the lowest in weight last. However, you still need to check in the 'Nutritional information' section of the label to be absolutely clear about the actual amount of the ingredient included. For example, salt may be last on the list of ingredients, but there could still be a hefty amount of salt, so it's necessary to check with the nutritional information given to find out the exact quantity. It will also give you the percentage figure (weight in grams per 100 grams). Some typical contents of a label are shown in Figure 4.1 – in this example they are for a cheese and tomato pizza.

NUTRITIONAL INFORMATION

Overall weight 405 g/14 oz

TYPICAL VALUES (when cooked)	Per ¼ pizza	Per 100 g
Energy	1102 kJ 262 kcal	1088 kJ 259 kcal
Protein	11.5 g	11.4 g
Carbohydrate of which sugars	30.2 g 1.6 g	29.8 g 1.6 g
Fat of which saturates	10.7 g 6.0 g	10.6 g 5.9 g
Fibre	3.6 g	3.6 g
Salt of which sodium	0.8 g 0.3 g	0.8 g 0.3 g
Per pizza ¼	262 calories	10.7 g fat

INGREDIENTS
Wheat flour, water, mozzarella cheese (21%), Cheddar cheese (9%), tomato, vegetable oil (including hydrogenated vegetable oil), yeast, flavouring, salt, sugar, herbs, flour treatment agent with dextrose emulsifier, E472(e), antioxidants, ascorbic acid, black pepper, puréed garlic.

Figure 4.1 An example of a food label

According to the British Heart Foundation guidelines (below page 25), this pizza has a 'middle range' fat and salt content per portion – in this case, a quarter of the pizza. However, if you try our home-made pizza (see pages 156–7), this will offer you even healthier levels of fat and salt per portion, without any added salt or sugar, without the cholesterol-raising hydrogenated oil (see page 10) and without the food additives.

One aspect of the food label you may find puzzling is that the values in the 'per 100 g' column – that is, the percentage column – only add up to 56.2 g, or 56.2 per cent, when you might expect it to add up to 100 g, or 100 per cent. This is because the water content of the pizza is not included in the calculations. However, it is included in the list of ingredients, coming after wheat flour in weight order.

So, water is clearly a major constituent of the pizza – a fact that is hardly surprising when you consider that our own bodies are composed of about 70 per cent water! By subtracting the percentage weight of the items listed on the nutritional label – 56.2 per cent from 100, we can calculate that the remaining 43.8 per cent of the pizza must, therefore, represent the water content. This provides the solution to the conundrum of the missing percentage figures.

How to make use of the information

As far as heart health is concerned, the most important items to examine on food labels are *energy*, *fat*, *sugar* (listed under *carbohydrate*) and *salt*.

Energy

The information on energy is provided in *kcal*, or *kilocalories*, and you will also find the metric equivalent information, given in *kilojoules, kJ*.

It depends on the amount of energy a person expends each day, of course, but an average, active woman may require 2000 kcals (8400 kJs) and an average, active man 2500 kcals (10,500 kJs) per day. It is also recommended that only about 30 to 35 per cent of total calories should come from *fat* and not more than a third of this from saturated fat. If we take the lower limit of 30 per cent, this means that someone with a 2000 kcals intake would be recommended to consume just around 67 g of total fat per day with 22 g of this being saturated fat. (These figures are arrived at by calculating 30 per cent of 2000 and then dividing the result by 9 – the energy equivalent in kcals of 1 g fat.) On the same basis, a person with a 2500-kcal intake would have a limit of 83 g of total fat per day, of which 28 g could be saturates. Current Government recommendations use a midpoint 33 per cent of calories (rather than 30 or 35 per cent) as the basis for the calculations, then round the figures down for women and up for men. So you'll find the recommended total fat targets listed on food products are 70 g fat for a woman with a 2000 kcals intake and 95 g for a man with a 2500 kcals intake. These are average figures, of course, and someone who is very active will need more calories than someone who is relatively inactive.

Fat

This is where it becomes important to be aware of the amount of fat in the food that we eat. For example, if the 'average' man eats a ready-made dish containing 35 g fat per portion, he will have used up just under 40 per cent of his recommended total of 95 g fat for that day, and a woman will have used half her recommended 70 g intake. Similarly, it's amazing how many calories can be consumed when using cooking or spreading fats. For example, it's not uncommon for people to spread 10–15 g margarine on a single slice of toast!

It's also crucial to be aware of how much hidden fat is to be found in shop-bought foods – in certain varieties of biscuits, crisps, puddings and cakes, for example. Some small (25-g) packets of crisps, for example, contain around 10 g of fat, with over a third of this being saturated fat. Equally, just one typical chocolate biscuit can also contain something like 7 g of fat, mostly saturated, and over 10 g of added sugar.

However, the good news is that, if you hunt around and check the labels, you should be able to find biscuits with a much lower fat content and you can get traditional crisps with only about 5 g of fat and a very low percentage of saturates. There are also some special types of thin crisps with less than 1 g of total fat in a 25-g serving. As a general rule of thumb, in selecting food items for fat content, you can use what has been called 'traffic light' advice.

Fat traffic lights

These are guidelines for judging acceptable total fat content per portion of food.

- If the fat content is 20 g or more, it's generally considered to be high total fat for one item of food. On the other hand, if it's an item to be shared, say between two to four people, and the proportion of saturated fat per person is low, then it would be fine. In terms of *total* fat per portion, anything below 3 g represents a little fat.
- Our advice is aimed at people generally wishing to eat for a healthy heart, but if you have special dietary needs, you may need to adjust your traffic light directions according to your own specific requirements. To enable most people to make realistic choices without limiting the range too much, we suggest that portions with a total fat content of 10 g or under might be taken to represent the *green* light, for GO, and 20 g or more, the *red* light for STOP (see figure 4.2 on page 22) . In between 10 and 20 g, you just need to use your judgement, but, where possible, aim to

keep the *saturated* fat content nearer to 1 g than 5 g per portion as 1 g saturated fat per portion is considered a little and 5 g a lot.

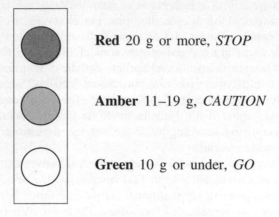

Red 20 g or more, *STOP*

Amber 11–19 g, *CAUTION*

Green 10 g or under, *GO*

Figure 4.2 Fat traffic lights

Sugar

As far as *sugar* is concerned, this is listed on food labels as a subdivision of carbohydrates. The only problem is that it's impossible at the moment to tell from the label how much of the sugar is intrinsic to the foods used in the product and how much is in the form of *added* or *free sugars*. These are defined by the World Health Organization as all the sugars added to foods or drinks by the manufacturer, cook or consumer, together with sugars naturally present in fruit juices, honey and syrups.

These added or free sugars contrast with the *unrefined* variety we consume when we eat fruit and vegetables. The unrefined sugar forms part of a highly nutritious food, full of valuable antioxidants, and this is generally considered to be the most beneficial form of sugar intake from a heart-health perspective. The sugar is bound up with the fruit and vegetable fibre and, because of this, is released into the bloodstream slowly. This means that it is much less likely than the quickly assimilated refined sugars to result in the sort of elevated levels of glucose and triglycerides that can lead to heart-related problems and diabetes.

Added or free sugars, however, are extracted from their source, refined and then used in processed foods and drinks or as packet sugar. They enter the bloodstream swiftly and need to be treated with some caution.

The inclusion of fruit juice in the added sugar category seems a little strange at first as fruit is one of the healthiest of food items. We need to remember, however, that these extracted juices often contain a high density of sugar and drinking such concentrated juice is not the same as eating a piece of raw fruit. This is why the generally accepted advice as mentioned earlier, is that, if you are using fruit juice as one of your daily five portions of fruit and vegetables, you should count only one small glass a day as one of these portions. It's also worth noting that a high intake of fruit juice (and other sugar-dense drinks) is related to poor dental health, particularly in children. If we overindulge in these drinks, the excess sugar will build up and be used by bacteria in the mouth, producing tooth-damaging acid that puts our teeth (and weight) at risk. So, enjoy the experience of drinking vitamin-rich fruit juices – they're good for you – but also check out the labels to see how much carbohydrate (sugar) they contain. If they're a bit high in sugar, you can dilute them with tap, mineral or carbonated water – all of which are sugar-free.

With respect to quantities, 10 g of added sugar – the equivalent of about 2 teaspoons of granulated sugar – is regarded as a large amount and 2 g as a little. The general advice is to try to keep on the low side. Unfortunately, as we have seen, food labels don't provide information about added sugars, making it difficult to calculate how much is contained in a particular item of processed food.

If you look at the pizza label (on page 19) for example, you will see that sugars are listed as a subdivision of the labelling information provided for carbohydrates. The figure 1.6 g for sugars is given for a portion (in this case, a quarter of the pizza) or 100 g. However, there is no way of telling how much of the sugar listed on a product like this is *intrinsic* to the other food ingredients involved (such as in the vegetables, which provide excellent overall health benefits) or *extrinsic* (added sugars), which require more careful scrutiny.

As far as the pizza is concerned, we know that this does contain added sugar because sugar is listed as the tenth ingredient by weight. What we don't know, though, is how much added sugar is involved. We think that it would be helpful to the consumer if food manufacturers were to provide an indication of the amount of added (free) sugar in their products. In the same way that fat is subdivided on the label to give the amount of saturated fat by using the phrase 'of which saturates', we consider that 'sugars' should be subdivided to give an amount for added sugar – 'of which added sugars'. For the moment, though, we have to guess by looking at where sugar is placed in the list of ingredients.

If an item contains below 5 g of sugar per portion overall (that is, including any added or free sugars), as in the case of the pizza we have been examining, then it's safe to assume that this is a reasonably healthy buy on the sugar front. With bought cakes and puddings, however, food manufacturers tend to include very high levels of sugar, often predominantly added sugar, so you'll have to look quite hard for suitable items here. Surprisingly, some low-fat ice-creams are considerably closer to recommended fat and sugar levels per portion than shop-bought cakes and puddings. Fortunately, as you will see from the Recipes section, there are plenty of appetizing puddings that keep both fat and sugar to acceptable limits and many of these can be made in less than 30 minutes. Others can be baked and frozen in portions to provide ready-made, healthy puddings for future occasions.

Salt

With salt, the best advice is to try to avoid using *additional* salt, because there is so much salt already included in processed foods. It is an essential mineral for the maintenance of good health, but most of us tend to have far too much in our diets and a high intake of salt is related to high blood pressure, which is one of the most important risk factors for heart disease and stroke.

You should try to keep your daily intake of salt *from all sources* below 7 g for men and 5 g for women. To help you calculate the amount of salt (sodium chloride) in a product when only the sodium content is provided, multiply the figure for sodium by 2.5. So, for example, 1 g of sodium per 100 g = 2.5 g of salt. On the pizza label there is 0.3 g of sodium per portion, which translates to 0.8 g of salt (0.3 x 2.5 = 0.75, which is then rounded up to 0.8 g).

Assessing the information

As a rough general rule of thumb when looking at fat, sugar and salt per 100-g portion, you can use Table 4.1 (adapted from the British Heart Foundation's leaflet, 'Guide to Food Labelling') to give you an idea of what constitutes a lot and what is a little.

Table 4.1 Guidelines for levels of sugar, fat and salt

	A lot	A little
Added sugar	10 g	2 g
Fat	20 g	3 g
saturates	5 g	1 g
Sodium	0.6 g	0.1 g
salt	1.5 g	0.3 g

Note: As the amounts of sodium in our recipes are low, the quantities in the Nutritional analyses are given in milligrams (1000 mg = 1 g). In the above table, under 'A little', for sodium the figure is 0.1 g, which would be 100 mg, and under 'A lot', 0.6 g sodium would be 600 mg.

For *daily* amounts of nutrients, Table 4.2 (adapted from the same British Heart Foundation leaflet) offers *rough* guidelines in relation to recommended calorie intakes for men and women, but remember that requirements will differ according to the amount of energy expended.

Table 4.2 Rough guidelines for daily intakes of nutrients

	Men	Women
Energy	2500 kcal	2000 kcal
Added sugars	70 g	50 g
Fat	95 g	70 g
Fibre	20 g	16 g
Salt	7 g	5 g

Drinks

As far as drinks are concerned, we mentioned earlier that wine with meals forms an enjoyable part of the healthy Mediterranean diet. The antioxidant flavonoids that wines (and other drinks such as tea and pomegranate or grape juice) contain help to protect against heart disease. However, it's important to follow the guidelines for sensible drinking because too much alcohol can damage your health. The recommended limits are expressed in units, where 1 unit is equivalent to:

- half a pint of ordinary strength beer, lager or cider
- a small 125-ml glass of wine, based on 11 per cent alcohol by volume (ABV on label)
- a single 25-ml pub measure of spirits (40 per cent ABV)
- a small, 50-ml glass of fortified wine, such as sherry, port, vermouth.

It takes our bodies between one to one-and-a-half hours (generally longer for women than men) to break down each unit of alcohol, and this is helped when consumption of alcohol is accompanied by food, as we've described in the Mediterranean-style diet.

The recommended maximum limits for the maintenance of good health are:

- no more than three to four units per day for men
- no more than two to three units for women
- and two alcohol-free days per week.

Most experts would suggest avoiding binge drinking and keeping to the lower rather than the higher limits in order to maintain maximum benefit and least risk to health.

Consumption of excessive amounts of any drink can be problematic, of course. Like alcoholic drinks, the content of many non-alcoholic beverages – especially the fizzy variety – are high in calories. One small, 330-ml can of cola, for example, might contain 33 g of sugar (that's around 7 teaspoons) and provide 135 kcal (567 kJ) of energy. So, for an average woman with a 2000 kcal intake per day, one can of cola will use up two-thirds of her maximum daily recommended amount of added sugar – 50 g or approximately 10 teaspoons. To use up the sugar contained in this one drink, she will need to expend a considerable amount of energy by taking physical exercise – perhaps half an hour's walk or a 15-minute jog. Without such energy use the calories will simply contribute to weight gain (see page 29).

There is also evidence to suggest that the sugars added to bought drinks (as with the sugar and fats in processed foods) can tend to become addictive. Fortunately, however, there are lots of delicious drinks (and foods) that don't contain large amounts of added sugar, but will quench our thirst and delight our palates without leading to potential problems with obesity (see pages 146–52).

In the next chapter we look at the relationship between intake of food and drink and output of energy and how to keep a healthy weight for a healthy heart.

5

Keeping a healthy weight
for a healthy heart

We're all born with certain tendencies, and some of these relate to our size and weight. There is also some evidence that our appetite levels are regulated by certain hormones and in some people, especially those with a tendency to become overweight, these hormone levels may be too low. Because of this such people do not feel full after eating and this may contribute to their overeating and, hence, to their weight problems. In the future, it may be possible to prescribe drugs to increase the levels of the relevant hormones, but such treatment will only be effective if accompanied by appropriate changes in lifestyle. Whatever our bodily make-up, we can largely determine to a considerable extent how fat we allow ourselves to become by choosing what we eat and how much exercise we take. It's largely a matter of matching our input of food and drink to our output in terms of physical activity – the more we eat, the more exercise we need to take. These issues are discussed in detail in the companion volume *How to Keep Your Cholesterol in Check*, but we will make one or two general points here.

By eating well and taking plenty of physical exercise we are helping our hearts to work better. We have seen how our choice of foods – keeping low on saturated fat especially – helps to determine the balance of highly desirable HDL cholesterol to the less desirable LDL. Well, physical exercise can help in the same way. It has the effect of increasing HDL cholesterol, lowering triglycerides and reducing the risk of developing coronary heart disease.

The best type of exercise for the heart muscle is the sort that increases your breathing rate and gets you slightly puffed – brisk walking, doing energetic housework or gardening, walking up and down stairs, swimming, cycling, playing badminton and so on. To get the most benefit for our hearts, the British Heart Foundation suggests that we should try to exercise like this for about 30 minutes on at least 5 days of the week, but any exercise will be beneficial. If you haven't been used to doing much physical exercise, it would be sensible to get yourself checked over by your GP or practice nurse before you start engaging in very vigorous exercise such as squash or half-marathons!

All sorts of physical exercise will help to use up calories gained by eating, as will activities our bodies carry out more or less automatically, such as breathing, digesting food, maintaining the brain, muscles and nerves in good working order and regulating temperature. If we eat too much for our needs and our calorie input becomes much greater than our energy output, however, we will put on weight.

One person complained about the expense of having to buy new clothes as her weight fluctuated: 'It's a good idea to try to keep in shape because I have to buy different clothes as I go up and down in size!' While becoming overweight can be costly in terms of clothes, it can be even more costly to health. Obesity is often an important contributing factor in the development of high blood pressure and heart disease. It is also one of the triggers for diabetes and there are an increasing number of people (and frequently nowadays young people) who develop diabetes as a result of being overweight. Mirroring trends in the USA (and to a lesser extent in Europe), a national audit on obesity in England found that nearly two-thirds of men and over half of women were overweight or obese – a fact that significantly increases the likely incidence of diseases such as diabetes and heart disease.

You can check your weight against a graph called a body mass index (BMI) chart. This gives you a rough guide to the appropriate weight for your height. It's not a perfect guide and doesn't make a distinction between men and women, whether you are active or inactive and it doesn't measure how much fat you are carrying. Even so, it is a useful guide and you can make your own estimate of your BMI by referring to Figure 5.1 on page 30.

Check-ups

If you think that you might be quite a bit overweight, it would be a good idea to arrange with your practice nurse at your GP's surgery to have a check-up. The nurse will be able to confirm your BMI and keep a check on your blood pressure. Doctors like to keep it no higher than about 150/90 mm Hg and the British Hypertension Society guidelines suggest that an optimal target should be 140/85 (the higher figure represents the maximum pressure the heart is using to pump blood round the body and the lower figure the minimum).

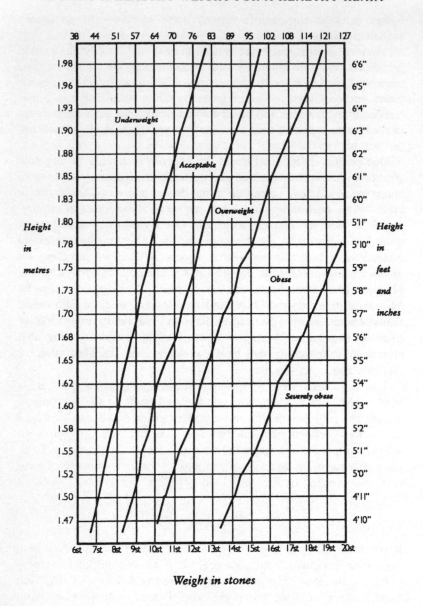

Figure 5.1 Body mass index (BMI) chart

When blood pressure starts to be persistently above this, your heart has to work harder than normal to push the blood through the arteries and, if this continues over a period of time, the heart can become enlarged. We can control blood pressure by a combination of eating healthy foods (keeping low on salt, for example), keeping a watch on weight and, where necessary, taking medication.

Your practice nurse will also be able to check the level of glucose in your urine or blood to make sure that you don't have a problem that can lead to diabetes. People who develop diabetes tend to have been born with a body chemistry that predisposes them to develop this problem, but it's not all down to our genes, as we have seen, and becoming overweight can result in the development of diabetes. You may have to ask for this, but, when you make an appointment to see the nurse, it would also be sensible to see if you can arrange for a fasting blood test to check on your total cholesterol and HDL cholesterol levels.

These checks, like an MOT you arrange for your car, will tell you what sort of nick you're in healthwise and this will guide you as to what sort of exercise it's reasonable for you to take, and what modifications, if any, you need to make to your diet in order to keep a healthy weight for a healthy heart. To help you in making any necessary changes, we have provided a few hints in Chapter 6.

6

Preparing for dietary change

People are often put off trying to change their diet because they
think it means giving up all the foods they most enjoy, but even
healthy eaters still enjoy tucking in to a good fish and chips from
time to time. And why not? An occasional treat is something we all
enjoy and it can be used by people who have to change their diets as
a sort of reward. In fact, if you are a fan of fish and chips, it's worth
noting that, with a bit of care in choosing and preparing the
ingredients, they can form the basis of an excellent low-fat meal! For
example, you can find low-fat oven chips in the supermarket that are
suitable even for people needing to keep saturates very low
(remember, there's less fat per chip in a 'chunky' rather than a 'thin'
chip). The fish can also be breaded and grilled, rather than fried, to
make a very acceptable and healthy meal for anyone. So, changing
our eating habits doesn't have to mean enjoying our food less and
many people have found that things taste much better with the new
approaches to buying and preparing food.

From time to time, we all find that we need to make changes to
our diet, whether it's to modify family meals to accommodate the
food fads of growing children or ageing parents, or to deal with
problems such as diabetes, or simply to try to eat more healthily.
This chapter focuses on the actual process of change.

Motivating yourself to change your diet

If I wanted to, then . . . if I had the motivation to do it, it would
probably be quite easy to change my diet . . . getting into a routine
and going shopping, getting the same things – but it's just making
that step really.

It's now considered that motivation to change our behaviour is
related to the number of perceived pros and cons associated with the
behaviour. For example, people may perceive changing to a healthy
diet to be 'good for the heart' – a pro – and this encourages them to
make changes, but they may also see it as 'boring and tasteless' – a
con – and this reduces their motivation to change. Usually when

people haven't made any serious attempt to change their behaviour – whether in relation to diet, smoking or drinking, for example – it's found that they imagine the cons of changing far outweigh the pros. Then, gradually, as they start thinking about changing, the numbers of pros increase until there seem to be more pros than cons and this is when change takes place. After this, we need to keep emphasizing the pros as we try to stick to the changes.

So, let's examine the evidence. We list below some of the cons and test the truth or falsehood behind a number of commonly held beliefs. Then we look at the pros.

The cons of eating a healthy diet

A friend of mine . . . he eats nothing else every day, all day, than Ryvita. Now personally I can't see what good it's doing him . . . I mean to eat Ryvita all day.

Fact

You don't have to eat only Ryvita to eat a healthy diet – in fact, restricting your diet in this sort of way is not a healthy option. There are many different foods that you can, and should, eat, as we have seen, and you don't have to rely on eating a number of specific 'healthy' foods to eat healthily. One of the keys to a balanced and healthy diet is to eat a *variety* of *different* foods.

My perception of what healthy eating would be like? Pretty boring, pretty bland . . . and really monotonous.

Fact

Healthy eating doesn't have to be boring or bland or monotonous, as we hope to show in the recipes included in this book. There is also now a broad range of tasty, low-fat and generally healthy foods available in the supermarkets. We just need to carry out our role as the canny food detective (see Chapter 4) to search out the products best suited to our individual needs.

Healthy eating would be more of an effort . . . you know, if you were to look round the supermarket for all the natural ingredients, things without additives, it'd take you a long time . . . much quicker and easier just to pick up a few frozen foods, frozen vegetables, stuff that's mass produced, probably with a pile of additives in them.

Fact

This may have been true a number of years ago, but nowadays supermarkets have made it easy for customers to shop for healthy foods. Food labels have become increasingly clearer to read (as we saw in Chapter 4), with some foods highlighted as healthy options. Some supermarkets even set whole sections aside as healthy choice zones. Also, don't be fooled, frozen foods and frozen vegetables are still healthy options. Vegetables and fruits retain many of their vitamins and minerals after they have been frozen and are a good replacement for fresh vegetables.

> It's the time factor. Things that take more than half an hour to prepare from start to finish, I might not bother ... I'd probably use convenience foods ... I think eating healthily often takes more preparation time.

Fact

Increasing numbers of healthy ready meals are now being manufactured and sold by supermarkets. These need very little preparation. Also, there are many healthy recipes that are quick and easy to prepare – see the Recipes section, 'Meals in under 30 minutes'.

> Well, I think to eat healthily ... if you really get the things that people say you should be getting, it's very, very expensive ... so I eat what my purse allows me to eat.

Fact

This is a common misperception that puts quite a few people off changing their eating habits, but healthy eating doesn't have to be any more expensive than unhealthy eating. In fact, in many cases the opposite is the case. Eating a wholly meat-based diet, with a high fat content, for example, is considerably more expensive than eating a largely vegetarian diet.

> I think it would be boring if you just ate the things that were good for you all the time, never having a good binge on burgers or sweets or ice-creams.

Fact

Even if you decide to change to a healthier diet, you can still eat the less healthy things sometimes. Rather than bingeing on them, though, it's important to try and eat them in smaller amounts and in moderation. Remember that once you have started to change your diet to a more healthy one, you'll almost certainly find that your tastes change, too, and you are not so often tempted by the items you always used to think of as 'naughty but nice': 'I used to have a really sweet tooth . . . and now I can't imagine how I managed to eat some of those yucky things.'

So, there are numerous cons that people perceive to be associated with healthy eating, often preventing them from changing to a healthy diet, but many of them are actually based on false beliefs. They should not stand in the way of any person who wants to start making a change and is willing to examine the evidence with an open mind.

The pros of eating a healthy diet

When I first decided to change my diet, I wasn't too sure it would do me any good, but now I can actually see the effects . . . my weight's gone down bit by bit, I'm more energetic and I just feel a lot better in myself. I'm really chuffed that I decided to stick to it.

Fact

In general, your weight is dependent on a balance between the amount of food you eat and the amount of energy you expend – for example, by exercising. Therefore, if you eat a healthier diet by reducing your fat intake and increasing your fruit, vegetable and fibre intake, while maintaining or slowly increasing your level of exercise, this should lead to a gradual, steady decrease in weight. This is generally recognized by dietitians as a good method of losing weight, as it is much easier to maintain the weight loss using this sort of approach than it is with faddy diets.

You get more vitamins through the vegetables and fruit and that should help with colds and infections and help you fight off things a bit more easily.

Fact

Eating for a healthy heart includes foods that contain many different vitamins and minerals. Intake of the necessary vitamins and minerals is important for the immune system, helping it to fight against various diseases. Also, diet has been found to have a key role in protection from illnesses such as heart disease, cancer and diabetes. Therefore, following a healthy diet should help to keep you healthy and protect you from both minor and major ailments.

Well, you feel better and you look better, I'm sure you do . . . all in all it's a sort of general well-being that you feel.

Fact

A fair amount of research now shows that what you eat is linked to the way you feel. That is, not only do our feelings influence the way we make certain food choices (for example, feeling stressed may lead us to eat chocolate) but also our food choices influence the way we feel. So, by eating healthily, we may also be helping to stimulate and maintain the feelings of physical and mental well-being that can so invigorate and refresh our daily living.

I'm sure that eating a balanced diet helps keep my energy levels up. It's probably the main thing that keeps me going like I do. When I used to binge on sweet stuff I'd get an immediate high, but it would wear off in no time and I'd soon feel absolutely knackered again!

Fact

Once we have eaten, our bodies convert the food into energy by means of a hormone called insulin. Sugary foods provide us with a quick release of energy, whereas other foods, such as wholemeal bread, wholemeal pasta, fruit and vegetables, provide us with energy that takes longer to break down and therefore lasts longer. So, eating healthily should create more of the long-lasting energy that will keep you going for longer.

Weighing up the pros and cons

It's clear, then, that there are quite a few pros associated with healthy eating. These are not only associated with your physical health but also your mental health or well-being – how you feel. It seems that healthy eating not only prevents disease but also gives you a better sense of well-being and more energy.

With all these pros, we should soon be able to fence off the cons and start the real business of making the changes.

7

Making dietary changes

If you're one of those people who has been thinking of changing your diet to benefit heart health, the next step is to make the changes and, when you have done this, to stick to them. This chapter offers you a number of practical tips to help start making the changes.

The following suggestions emerged from the research programme *The Nation's Diet*.

Do it gradually

It's usually easier to make changes gradually, rather than all at once, as this makes the process of adjustment easier. For example, if you are drinking full-fat milk at the moment, try cutting down on fat by switching to semi-skimmed and get used to that first before moving on to skimmed milk. Also, don't go for drastic solutions, such as cutting out fatty and sweet foods altogether. Cut down on them slowly and reduce your portions. Once you have started, you'll find you can gradually bring in and try out more of the healthy recipes, then leave out more of the less healthy ones. You'll also find that any craving for the less healthy foods gradually diminishes as your palate becomes more accustomed to your new, healthier eating style and you begin to enjoy the taste and variety of the new menus even more than the old.

Get support from other people

Get someone else who is close to you to eat healthily with you. It is much easier to keep yourself motivated if there is more than just you. The good news is that eating for a healthy heart is an accessible and enjoyable option for anybody, so getting someone else involved is good for both of you. It's not a strict, punishing dietary regime that is tasteless and boring – there's a whole range of tasty meals that you can prepare and we'll hope to tempt you to try them later. Enjoy choosing your menus together – it's so much easier than having to cook two separate dishes, one for your family or partner and one for yourself.

Find substitutes for 'unhealthy' foods and snacks

Saying 'no' to 'unhealthy' foods, such as the varieties of biscuits, cakes and crisps that are very high in hidden fat, is possibly one of the most difficult things you'll have to cope with because buying these foods may have become part of your regular shopping routine. It's not too difficult to find excellent substitutes, though, once you've identified the foods that you need to change – for example, apple or carrot slices instead of biscuits, or water biscuits instead of crisps. We're back to the food detectives again, finding out how much fat and sugar different items in your current shopping basket contain. However, once you've done this, you can enjoy the next step – searching out some really tasty substitutes.

For further help in making food substitutions, we have set out a number of suggested alternatives in Table 7.1 on page 39 that are beneficial to good heart health.

Don't put temptation in your way

A lock on the fridge has been suggested as the only effective guard against any tempting goodies within! A bit of an extreme suggestion, perhaps, which could raise complications if you're living with other people. One big help when making changes is to ensure that the fruit bowl and the kitchen cupboards are well stocked and the fridge and the freezer are full of the sort of foods that you've decided to change to, rather than the high-sugar, high-fat ones you're trying to leave behind. The best thing is not to buy those foods in the first place – leave them in the shops.

Have occasional treats

You don't have to give up all your indulgences for ever if you're trying to follow a healthy diet. It's important that you still have occasional treats. As long as you choose a balanced diet and don't indulge too often, then it is fine to treat yourself from time to time. Don't punish yourself afterwards – just enjoy it.

Table 7.1 Some suggested food substitutions

If you eat this	Try switching to
Breakfast	*Breakfast*
Sweetened cereal with full-fat milk	Home-made muesli (see pages 55–6), unsweetened cereal or porridge with skimmed or semi-skimmed milk and fruit
White toast and butter	Wholemeal or wholegrain toast and low-fat, unsaturated or plant stanol/sterol spread
Fried egg and bacon	Grilled lean bacon, poached egg and toast
Snack meals	*Snack meals*
Cheese or beefburger	Wholemeal bread sandwich with tuna or cottage cheese and chutney or grilled, low-fat vegeburger (Quorn or soya-based) in wholemeal roll
Pies and pasties	Lentil and tomato soup and wholemeal roll (see page 155)
Chips	Jacket potato and baked beans
Main meals	*Main meals*
Fried fish and chips	Grilled fish, new potatoes or low-fat oven chips and peas
Steak and kidney pie or shepherd's pie made with mince	Shepherd's pie made with soya, Quorn or lean mince
Fried sausage and deep-fried chips	Grilled sausage (made with Quorn, soya or lean meat), jacket potato or low-fat oven chips and baked beans
Meat stew and suet dumplings	Bean goulash and dumplings made with oil or unsaturated margarine (see pages 95–6)
Puddings	*Puddings*
Apple pie and cream	Low-fat blackberry and apple crumble made with oats and oil (see pages 119–20)
Rich cream gateau or cheesecake	Low-fat cheesecake (see pages 125–6)
Crème caramel	Low-fat milk pudding and dried fruit
Individual mousse	Low-fat yogurt or fromage frais with fruit
Extra snacks	*Extra snacks*
Doughnuts, pastries	Raisin malt loaf (see pages 139–40) teacakes
Biscuits high in hidden fat	Water biscuits, Ryvita, wholemeal or wholegrain bread or toast or currant and red wine biscuits (see pages 136–7)
Cheese and biscuits	Fresh fruit
Chocolates, sweets, crisps	Carrots, fresh and dried fruit, nuts (often regarded as off the menu because of their high fat content, but see pages 55–6)

8
Maintaining the changes

Once you have managed to make changes to your diet, it then becomes important to try to stick to them, so that the benefits to health and fitness will also be maintained. The challenge now is how to keep determined and motivated. The rest of this chapter provides a few tips on maintaining dietary changes.

Keep reminding yourself why you decided to change

Don't let yourself forget why you decided to make the changes to your diet. Remember any times when being overweight made you feel uncomfortable – perhaps being unable to run for buses or walk without becoming short of breath. Remind yourself of all the positive things that you are gaining from eating healthily. Think back to the negative things you thought would be part of eating healthily and note how few of these have turned out to be true.

Remember how much evidence there is linking good diet to good health

Although you will probably feel fitter and healthier because of your new eating habits, it's possible that you may not feel any immediate physical advantages. If this happens, remind yourself of the growing amount of research that demonstrates the indisputable link between poor diet and the long-term development of disease. Enjoy eating healthy foods and the delicious recipes you've been preparing in the knowledge that your efforts are helping your body to remain healthy and resist disease.

You could also check on spending patterns. You should notice that your spending on food hasn't gone through the roof as you thought it might. In fact, you might even find that you are spending less!

Don't be put off by initial problems in changing your diet

Although at first the changes will seem different and new to you, before long you will get into a routine and this will make it easier for you to stick to your diet. You'll find that you will be picking up the same sorts of foods each time you go shopping (much as you did before, only the foods will be different). You'll also be getting into a new routine with cooking and preparing food. After a short time, the changes to your lifestyle will no longer feel different, but will be integrated into your daily routine.

Don't worry if you can't always stick to your changed diet

Some days it may be easier to stick to your eating plans than others. Often people find, for example, that it's harder to keep motivated if they're feeling a bit down or depressed. Then it seems much easier to give up and grab a treat for comfort. There are a number of ways of coping with such situations.

First, if you have decided not to have certain foods, such as chocolate biscuits or cream cakes in your house, you are less likely to treat yourself as they are not so readily available. Second, before eating a large cream cake, for example, stop for a moment to imagine how you'll feel after you have eaten it. Would you feel healthier and pleased with yourself or less healthy and cross with yourself? Often people who turn to foods for comfort feel considerably worse after they have binged rather than better. Try to think of the potentially uncomfortable after-effects before you indulge.

Finally, if it's all too much and you end up giving in to a cream cake or a large bar of chocolate, don't punish yourself for days afterwards. This won't really help; it will just make you more miserable. So, treat it as a one-off and continue with your healthy eating plan. It's not bad or wrong to have the odd treat. An occasional planned treat is to be encouraged and an unscheduled one is just a momentary blip!

9

Dealing with tricky situations

Being invited to lunch or dinner at a friend's house can be potentially embarrassing if you're trying to stick to a low-fat diet or you're vegetarian, because of the extra constraints this places on the person providing the meal. Of course, the best way to deal with these sorts of situations is to speak to the person beforehand if you can and give some examples of what is on or off the menu for you. Although this can feel awkward, it's much easier tackling the problem before the meal rather than when you've arrived and you're left with very little option but to eat what is put in front of you!

Canteens

Many work or college canteens produce very nutritious and healthy foods, but there are still some that have not taken on board the basics of healthy eating. One woman called some of the meals produced by these places 'heart disease on a plate', where the fat was 'just running off'! If your canteen does not offer healthy meals, try asking if they could provide some of your own favourite, healthier alternatives or take your own sandwiches – at least you know what ingredients have gone into them and you can ensure that you have a healthy option available. Home-made sandwiches are also often much cheaper and tastier than bought ones.

What about Christmas?

Once again, don't worry about having the occasional day off from healthy eating. However, there are healthy options at Christmas – check out the healthy Christmas pudding on pages 118–19.

Will the children make a fuss?

Cooking for a family is, of course, more difficult than cooking just for you, but here are a few general points that might help:

- if you decide to try new foods, introduce them along with old favourites

- make changes simply, slowly and one at a time
- concentrate on making mealtimes an enjoyable experience
- introduce a healthy diet for the whole family from the beginning if possible – good habits start early
- get your children involved in choosing, planning and preparing meals and in shopping for their favourite recipes
- emphasize the relationship between healthy eating and looking and feeling in good shape.

Very young children and a low-fat diet

Children under the age of two shouldn't have low-fat milk – they haven't developed big enough stomachs at this age to cope with a lot of low-energy, high-fibre foods, so they need full-fat milk to provide enough energy for growth. If they're over two years old, they can have semi-skimmed milk and, from the age of five, skimmed milk. From the age of five they can (and should) enjoy the same healthy foods as adults following the general principles outlined in this book.

Does a vegetarian or vegan diet provide all the right sorts of nutrients?

Most vegetarian diets are absolutely fine for the whole family. You just have to make sure that the diet you choose is well balanced and contains all the necessary nutrients. Fortunately, you can get a whole range of nutrients from fruit and vegetables (including pulses), from a variety of Quorn and soya products and from bread, pasta, rice, cereals and nuts. All these vegetarian options also have a low fat content, apart from nuts. However, as we have seen, much of the fat in nuts tends to be monounsaturated and this actually helps to reduce cholesterol levels. So, even the higher-fat nuts are heart healthy.

People on vegetarian diets sometimes worry that, because they don't eat meat, they won't get enough iron. It's true that meat is a good source of this nutrient, but iron can also be found in eggs, pulses, dried fruit, dark green leafy vegetables and iron-enriched breakfast cereals, so it really isn't a problem. A useful tip is to remember that orange juice helps our bodies to absorb iron from the food we eat. While you are enjoying a refreshing glass of orange juice, you're also helping your body to increase its intake of iron.

If you are a vegan and do not eat any food from animal sources, one of the few tricky bits is ensuring that you're getting enough vitamin B12, but you'll find that lots of cereals have this added to them, especially Grapenuts, yeast extract and fortified soya milk (though check the label). Fortified soya milk can also provide an extra source of calcium for vegans, in addition to that obtained from dried fruit, dark green leafy vegetables, sesame seeds and nuts.

In general, then, following a vegetarian diet is a healthy option and some research suggests that non-meateaters tend to have less heart disease (and cancer) than meateaters.

Eating out

It's probably best to regard eating out as one of those special occasions when you just enjoy the food and company without worrying too much about the ingredients in the dishes. If, however, you eat out regularly on a social or work basis or you have to keep a close check on your intake of fat, sugar or salt, eating out may need extra care. Even then, it can still remain a pleasure and not a nightmare if you follow the few simple guidelines we set out in the next chapter.

10

Eating out on a low-fat diet

It can be hard to settle for 'just a salad' when everyone else around you is choosing scrumptious, but high-fat, dishes. A lot of the food on offer in restaurants, cafés and takeaways is likely to be higher in saturated fat, sugar and salt than the food you eat at home. So, be prepared to choose items that fit in with your own dietary requirements and don't be afraid to ask about ingredients and cooking methods. Most good restaurants are proud of what they cook and will be happy to advise you. Eventually you will know the restaurants that can provide you with the delicious food you want to eat – and that shouldn't just mean salads!

Useful tips for eating out if you are on a special, reduced-fat diet

- Plan ahead. Consider what you will be eating later in the day and choose a lunch to balance that out.
- Take the edge off your hunger before you go out – have some fruit, say – to stop you ordering a big meal because you're ravenous.
- Take some plain bread from the bread basket but decline the butter. Ask for extra bread and try different varieties.
- Choose only a two-course meal and ensure that at least one is based on vegetables, seafood or fruit.

When choosing from the menu, here are some suggestions for keeping low on fat.

- Simple low-fat starters include melon, chilled fruit juice or salads with a little olive oil dressing.
- Choose a vegetable-based soup, such as carrot and coriander, minestrone or leek and potato, with a crusty bread roll. Avoid creamy soups.
- Choose plenty of vegetables with your main course – without sauces or butter. Portion sizes are often bigger than you would have at home, so you could ask for half a portion of the main course with a double portion of vegetables or salad.

- Avoid salads with mayonnaise dressings. Ask for a little olive oil, vinegar or oil-free dressing.
- Go for dishes that are steamed, braised, grilled, chargrilled or baked. Avoid anything fried, sautéed, battered or smothered in cheese or a cream sauce as it is likely to be very high in fat. Ask for sauces to be served in separate dishes so that you can control the amount of sauce that you put on your food.
- Don't assume that vegetarian dishes are always the best choice – check on the fat content first. Do choose dishes based on beans and other pulses with pasta, rice, potatoes, bread and extra vegetables and salads. Avoid pastry and too much cheese.
- Boiled or steamed new potatoes, jacket potatoes, plain pasta and rice are better choices than sautéed or roast potatoes or chips.
- Ask for a jug of water or bottle of mineral water. Although alcoholic and sugary drinks will not contribute to your fat intake, they will certainly bump up the calories.
- For a dessert, go for a fresh fruit salad, exotic fresh fruit, sorbets or fruit yogurts.
- Ask for milk with your tea or coffee – not cream.

Fast food

If you're following a diet with a restricted fat intake, but you like to visit your local burger bar or you fancy picking up a snack during your lunchbreak from a baker or supermarket, here are some ideas.

- Choose a grilled chicken, vegetarian or fish burger or plain hamburger and avoid the cheese.
- Order a smaller (child's portion) hamburger to reduce the fat.
- Steer clear of mayonnaise.
- Order a baked jacket potato instead of a burger and avoid added butter – go for toppings such as baked beans, tuna without mayonnaise, vegetable chilli or curry or cottage cheese instead – and order a side salad.
- Go for sandwiches or baguettes with, for example, tuna and salad without mayonnaise, rather than pasties and pies.

As far as eating out at other restaurants is concerned, here are a few tips that are worth considering if you have been advised to keep to a low-fat diet.

Indian restaurants

It's not particularly easy to find very low-fat dishes in Indian restaurants or takeaways because of the tendency for food to be deep-fried, and ghee, the Indian cooking fat, has a similar amount of saturated fat as butter. Here, though, are some suggestions to help reduce the fat content.

- Choose the drier dishes, such as tandoori, karahi and bhuna, spinach-based ones (saag) and chicken tikka dishes.
- Choose dishes with saffron and plain boiled rice rather than pilau, biriyani or fried rice, which tend to be high in fat.
- Enjoy side dishes such as yogurt raita.
- Choose chapattis or naan breads. Avoid breads made with fat, such as peshwari, paratha and puris.
- Choose grilled poppadums if available (not fried).
- Choose rogan josh and jalfrezi dishes – both have tomato-based sauces and are, therefore, healthier options than some of the others on offer.
- Vegetable dishes, such as aloo gobi, a potato and cauliflower curry, can be reasonably low in fat, but check that they're not cooked in ghee.
- Try to avoid creamy dishes, such as korma, masala and dhansak, and oily ones, such as bhajis, samosas or pakhoras. Also, check for the ghee in dupiaza, madras and vindaloo dishes.

Chinese restaurants

- Choose chicken and sweetcorn, sweetcorn and crab or won ton soup rather than pancake rolls for starters.
- Chicken with beansprouts, chilli prawns or crab, steamed crab with spring onions and ginger are good choices.
- Choose plain boiled or steamed rice. Avoid fried rice, prawn crackers and sesame prawn roll.
- Choose stir-fried dishes rather than deep-fried ones, such as stir-fried vegetables, chicken or beef in black bean sauce. Sweet and sour and crispy fried dishes, such as crispy fried duck, are best avoided because of their high fat content. Satay and chow mein dishes are a little less fatty than these, but they're still best considered as special treats.

Japanese and Thai restaurants

- Stir-fried dishes cooked in small amounts of hot oil don't absorb much fat, but deep-fried items do, such as spring rolls.
- Enjoy the variety of vegetables available with plenty of plain rice.
- It's difficult to avoid coconut milk in Thai food, which contains much saturated fat, but the good news is that it may not be as harmful to heart health as previously thought. A report from the World Health Organization (WHO), 'Diet, Nutrition and the Prevention of Chronic Diseases' (2003), concluded that there is likely to be less potential risk to heart health from lauric acid (the main fatty acid in coconut) than from the trans-fatty acids, palm oil and saturated fats contained in food from animal sources, for which the evidence of a relationship with poor heart health is clear and convincing. However, if you do want to use coconut milk in your cooking, it is still sensible to look out for the reduced-fat varieties or dilute with water.
- Chicken and seafood are good choices – lamb and pork are higher in fat.

Italian restaurants

- Choose vegetable and fruit starters or bean soup with breadsticks or plain crusty bread rather than garlic bread, which can be very high in fat. If you're cooking at home, however, try our recipe for Garlic toasties, given on page 54.
- Enjoy mixed or tomato salads with only a tiny splash of dressing.
- Choose thin-crust pizza with vegetables, ham, chicken, tuna, Hawaiian or seafood toppings. These pizzas tend to be less calorific and fatty than deep-pan pizzas with other meats and toppings. Avoid high-fat meats, such as salami or pepperoni, and too much cheese, for example.
- Choose pasta with tomato-based or seafood sauces – arrabbiata sauce (tomato and chilli), for instance. Avoid rich, creamy sauces or those with large amounts of cheese or pesto. A little grated Parmesan cheese on top will give flavour without adding too much fat.
- Dishes such as lasagne and spaghetti bolognese can have a very high fat content. Some lasagnes contain more fat than a plate of fish and chips! So, we offer you low-fat versions of each (pages 98–100; 157–8). When eating out, cannelloni is often a better choice as a major part of the dish tends to consist of spinach.

Mexican restaurants

- Good choices are spicy corn chowder and black bean soups.
- Fill up on Mexican rice and vegetable chilli.
- Chicken fajitas or Cajun chicken are likely to be reasonably low in fat, but beware enchiladas – these have a high fat content (but see our low-fat recipe on pages 88–9).
- Tomato-based salsa sauces and dips are generally fine, but avoid sour cream. See the Recipes section for a low-fat home-made salsa dip (page 67).
- Choose gazpacho.
- Guacamole and refried beans are a mixed bag as they contain a lot of cardioprotective nutrients but they are also high in fat, so take it steady. However, do try our low-fat Guacamole recipe on page 57.

So, even those on medically supervised low-fat diets can still enjoy a wide variety of foods from all over the world, safe in the knowledge that they are still eating for a healthy heart. Just follow our guidelines.

11
Ten healthy eating tips

I think eating a properly balanced, mixed diet affects the kind of person you are in personality, in health and in outlook ... you know, with a spring in your step, rather than the lethargic cartoon sitting on the couch with a bag of crisps and a beefburger kind of thing ... I think it makes you more alive.

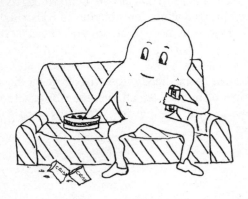

Here are ten suggestions to help you keep that spring in your step!

- Make sure you aim for a balanced diet in which you eat a variety of nutritious foods, with your meals spread through the day, and keep to moderately sized food portions.
- Keep low on salt and fats, especially saturated fat. Instead, choose unsaturated fats and oils wherever possible and keep an eye on the hidden fats and salt, such as those in biscuits and processed foods.
- Get plenty of exercise to sharpen your appetite and give your heart, lungs and blood vessels a regular workout.
- Aim to avoid becoming apple-shaped, but do eat plenty of apples and other fruit and vegetables (at least five portions a day) plus some nuts – all high in antioxidants.
- Lower triglycerides and blood pressure, increase HDL cholesterol and prevent your blood getting too sticky by eating oily fish at least once a week.

- Don't kill off the heart health benefits of your good diet by smoking, which accounts for about a third of deaths from coronary heart disease and stroke and is the cause of most cancers of the lung, trachea, larynx, mouth and oesophagus. The companion volume *How to Keep Your Cholesterol in Check* gives advice on how to stop smoking.
- Eat plenty of wholemeal bread, potatoes, rice and pasta, cereals (such as oats) and pulses (beans and so on).
- Try skimmed or semi-skimmed instead of full-fat milk and limit your intake of high-fat cheese.
- Grill, use a wok, steam or microwave rather than deep fry.
- Try cooking the Mediterranean way, with olive oil, garlic and plenty of fresh vegetables. Eat at a leisurely pace, enjoy your glass of wine and relax!

Now it's your turn

We have set out in the remaining pages a range of recipes that we hope will give you good starting points for the development of your own individual approaches to eating for a healthy heart. All the recipes are designed with your heart in mind, so you will find, for example, that we have kept low on fat and sugar, sometimes avoiding added fat completely by using replacements, as in the use of a prune or apricot purée in Grandma's favourite fruit cake (page 143). When using milk, we have used skimmed milk for the most part, but you could interchange with semi-skimmed or soya milk, according to preference. Where fat is used for cooking, we have used predominantly monounsaturated or polyunsaturated oil or margarine (described in the recipes as 'unsaturated margarine'). You need to check that the margarine is suitable for baking, as some aren't, but you can get some very good low-salt, low-fat versions (less than 60 per cent fat) that work very well and we have used these to calculate the nutritional figures. We don't think you will find that using these unsaturated varieties of fat will have a detrimental effect as far as the taste of the food is concerned, but if some of you do find that the recipes are not quite to your liking initially, then modify them slightly. Even people who are changing from quite high-fat/high-sugar foods to the ones with lower concentrations we have recommended will gradually find that their palates become educated to the new tastes so that they begin to relish their new-style meals as much (and often more) than they did the versions they ate in the past. Healthy eating shouldn't be a penance; it should be a pleasure. Just think of all those delicious foods that are available in plenty and are actually doing you good – providing you with all the healthy nutrients you require to keep your heart and body in good shape and to resist disease.

The latest edition of the companion volume, *How to Keep Your Cholesterol in Check*, also by Dr Robert Povey, contains a handful of recipes especially suitable for people with cholesterol problems. These have been included in the present book, together with one or two recipes that have already appeared in the monthly *H·E·A·R·T UK Digest* (formerly *The Family Heart Digest*), but more than 90 per cent of the recipes have been designed and developed specifically for this book.

Where a recipe includes meat, we have also suggested a vegetarian alternative – Quorn or soya products such as tofu or textured vegetable protein (TVP) instead of meat.

All the recipes have been checked by a specialist dietitian, Jacqui Morrell. They are full of heart-healthy ingredients and, as far as fat content is concerned, each recipe is within the green light for 'go', with 10 g or less fat per serving (see pages 21–2).

We hope that you enjoy trying out the recipes. Don't regard them as carved in stone, though – play about with them and use them as a basis for producing your own imaginative (and healthy) party pieces. Eating for a healthy heart shouldn't be dull and boring; it should be exciting, satisfying, tasty and, above all, a thoroughly enjoyable experience. Bon appetit!

Recipes

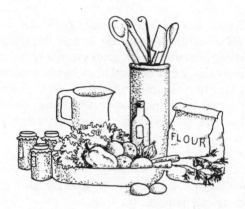

Starters and snacks

Garlic toasties
Serves 2–4

The garlic bread you get in restaurants often has a very high fat content, so for a version without the excess fat, try these delicious Garlic toasties as a starter or as soup croûtons.

Did you know that garlic cloves, like onions, leeks and chives, are full of heart-healthy properties? They are rich in antioxidants and can benefit your health in many ways. Garlic has also been shown to help keep bacteria at bay, lower blood pressure and bad LDL cholesterol levels while tending to increase the good HDL.

Ingredients
1 garlic clove   2 tsp olive oil
2 large slices of wholemeal
    bread

Nutritional analysis
Per toast finger, 18 kcals (76 kJ), 1 g fat, of which negligible saturates, 33 mg sodium.

Method
1 Crush the garlic and mix with the oil.
2 Place the bread slices on a piece of kitchen foil and spread the oil and garlic mixture over both sides of the bread.
3 Grill gently, 3 or 4 minutes for each side until nicely browned. You need to keep a close eye on them to make sure that they don't burn.
4 Cut into 12 toast fingers and serve as a Garlic toasty starter or cut into smaller pieces and use as croûtons.

Bagels
Serves 1

Bagels are popular for breakfast, brunch, lunchboxes and a pick-me-up snack.

They are low in fat and are good with a variety of fillings. Here are some ideas that you could also use with ordinary bread rolls, baguettes or pitta bread:

- sliced bananas and raisins
- low-fat cheese spread and smoked salmon
- chicken or turkey and salad
- ricotta cheese and tomatoes
- peanut butter and watercress
- hard-boiled egg, fromage frais and cress
- reduced-fat cheese and beetroot
- lean bacon, lettuce and tomato
- sardines and tomato
- tuna and sweetcorn.

Nutritional analysis
Per bagel, 260 kcals (1092 kJ), negligible fat and 250 mg sodium.

Home-made muesli
Makes 450 g (1 lb), 15 x 30-g (1-oz) servings

Oats (especially oat bran) are particularly good at lowering total cholesterol levels. Try an oat-based muesli for breakfast with skimmed, semi-skimmed or soya milk. As a light dessert, add some to yogurt or just munch as a snack. There are lots of muesli mixes around or you can make your own by adding dried fruit with perhaps a few vitamin-fortified bran flakes and nuts to a base of oats.

Dried fruits, such as sultanas and raisins, are excellent ingredients for muesli. You can add other fruits, too – grapes, apricots or prunes – for a good antioxidant munch.

Nuts are also especially valuable in a heart-healthy diet. They provide an excellent food source for vitamin E and selenium and help to reduce cholesterol. Although generally quite high in fat, they contain very little saturated fat, apart from coconut which is high in saturates (but see Chapter 10, under 'Japanese and Thai restaurants' on page 48, for more details on how coconut may be less harmful to the heart than previously believed).

Hazelnuts, almonds and pecan nuts are predominantly mono-unsaturated (with less than 10 per cent saturates), as are cashew and Brazil nuts (but these have twice as much saturated fat). Walnuts, pine nuts and sunflower seeds, on the other hand, have predominantly polyunsaturated fat (90 per cent). Some nuts also contain omega-3 fats (walnuts and pecan nuts, for example), and flax seeds (linseed) are especially rich in these beneficial fatty acids.

We suggest a possible combination of ingredients, but this is just a single possibility out of 1001 or more, so over to you!

Ingredients

200 g (7 oz) oats
55 g (2 oz) oat bran
40 g ($1\frac{1}{2}$ oz) bran flakes
100 g ($3\frac{1}{2}$ oz) mixed dried fruit

55 g (2 oz) mixed nuts – half walnuts and half hazelnuts, roughly chopped, make a nice mix

Nutritional analysis

Per 30-g (1-oz) serving, 114 kcals (479 kJ), 4 g fat, of which saturated fat negligible, 33 mg sodium.

Method

1 Place all the ingredients in a plastic container, seal with lid and shake well to mix. Serve with skimmed, semi-skimmed or un-sweetened soya milk. Also delicious with yogurt and fruit.

Other easy ways to eat more seeds and nuts

- Use toasted cashews or sesame seeds in a chicken or Quorn or tofu stir-fry, and top a fruity dessert with toasted almonds.
- Spread bread with peanut butter or tahini rather than margarine.
- Sprinkle a mixture of mixed nuts and linseeds (flax seeds) over cereal or salads, or add to baked foods like muffins.

Guacamole
Serves 4

For this recipe, the avocado needs to be ripe. To check this, press the base – if it's hard and doesn't give, allow it to ripen for a couple of days before using.

Although avocados are high in fat, about 80 per cent of the fat is unsaturated and over 60 per cent is monounsaturated, so it's 'good' fat. Avocados also provide an excellent supply of vitamin E, potassium and folic acid. They contain a cholesterol-lowering plant sterol called beta-sitosterol – overall, a very heart-healthy food.

Ingredients

1 ripe avocado
1 large tomato, diced
1 shallot, finely chopped
4-cm ($1\frac{1}{2}$-in) piece cucumber, diced

$\frac{1}{4}$ tsp chilli powder
dash Tabasco sauce
freshly ground black pepper
juice of $\frac{1}{2}$ lemon

Nutritional analysis

Per serving, 81 kcals (340 kJ), 7 g fat, of which 2 g saturated, 28 mg sodium.

Method

1 Halve the avocado and remove the stone. Scoop out the avocado flesh into a bowl using a spoon and pour the lemon juice over it. Add the tomato, shallot and cucumber and mash together lightly to make a chunky mixture. Finally, add the chilli powder and Tabasco and season with pepper.
2 Chill for 15–20 minutes in the fridge.
3 Serve with toast or tortilla chips. The latter can be a bit high in fat, but a handful (say 6 or so) should only add about 2 g fat to your starter, so just enjoy them!

Hummus
Serves 4–6

Delicious with pitta bread, crudités, toast fingers or just as a sandwich filling. To keep the fat content down, we have reduced the amount of olive oil. This makes it a little thicker and less oily in texture than the traditional recipe, but produces a really tasty dish. If you want to increase the quantity, just use more chickpeas and stock.

You can speed up the preparation time by using cooked, tinned chickpeas, but remember that the 115 g (4 oz) dried chickpeas in the recipe will double in weight when cooked. So, look at the 'drained weight' on the tin and make sure that this is roughly twice the weight of the dried chickpeas in the recipe. Also, rather than using the salty liquid from the tin as stock, substitute water.

Ingredients
115 g (4 oz) dried chickpeas, soaked overnight
1 garlic clove, left whole
8–9 tbsp liquid from cooking chickpeas
2 level tbsp tahini
1 tsp extra virgin olive oil
juice of 1 lemon
$\frac{1}{4}$ tsp paprika
freshly ground black pepper
2 sprigs fresh parsley, chopped, to garnish

Nutritional analysis
For 4 servings, per serving, 158 kcals (664 kJ), 8 g fat, of which 1 g saturated, 13 mg sodium. For 6, each provides 105 kcals (441 kJ), 5 g fat, of which 1 g saturated, 9 mg sodium.

Method
1 Drain and rinse the chickpeas. Place in a large pan with plenty of fresh water. Add the garlic, bring to the boil and boil rapidly for 10 minutes. Reduce the heat, cover and simmer until the chickpeas are soft. This will take 1–1$\frac{1}{2}$ hours. Drain thoroughly, reserving the liquid.
2 Place 8 tablespoons of the reserved liquid, the chickpeas, tahini, lemon juice and olive oil into a food processor. (If you particularly like the taste of raw garlic, add an extra crushed clove to the ingredients at this stage.) Mix to a thick paste. Add more of the reserved liquid if necessary. Season with the paprika and black pepper.
3 Spoon the hummus into a dish and garnish with the chopped parsley.

Vegetable samosas
Makes 4

Samosas cooked in restaurants or bought in supermarkets can be a bit on the fatty side, so why not try making your own? In this version, we use low-fat filo pastry to wrap the delicious, spicy vegetable ingredients.

Serve with Mango chutney (pages 70–1) or a raita (chopped cucumber and fresh mint mixed with natural yogurt) as a tasty starter or accompaniment to an Indian meal.

The Samosas freeze well. Simply follow steps 1 to 5 of the Method, freeze, then defrost when you want to use them and reheat on the middle shelf of a preheated 180°C (350°F/gas mark 4) oven for 10 minutes.

Ingredients

1 tsp olive oil (or spray), plus extra for greasing
1 shallot, finely chopped
2 medium (170 g (6 oz) each) sweet potatoes, diced (about 1-cm ($\frac{1}{2}$-in) cubes)
1 medium carrot, diced
50 g (2 oz) frozen peas

1 level tsp garam masala
$\frac{1}{4}$ tsp chilli powder
1 tbsp fresh coriander, chopped
1 tsp fresh mint, chopped
juice of 1 lime
freshly ground black pepper
2 sheets filo pastry

Nutritional analysis
Per Samosa, 153 kcals (643 kJ), 2 g fat, of which saturated fat negligible, 175 mg sodium.

Method
1 Lightly grease a baking tray, preheat the oven to 180°C (350°F/ gas mark 4), then place (or spray) a little of the oil in a large frying pan or flameproof casserole. Add the vegetables, cover and cook for about 10 minutes over a very low heat, tossing and turning the vegetables occasionally to prevent burning and to ensure that they are evenly cooked.

2 Stir in the dry spices. Add the fresh coriander and mint, then pour in the lime juice. Cook for 2 minutes. Season to taste with black pepper.

3 Cut each filo pastry sheet in half lengthways and lay on a floured surface. Spoon a quarter of the mixture on to the end of one halved sheet of filo. It will look like quite a lot of mixture, but

keep going. Take hold of one of the corners and fold the pastry over the mixture so that it is enclosed and the top layer of the filo sheet now forms a triangle. Then take hold of the point at the other end corner and fold the filo pastry triangle over, and continue folding in triangles in this way until you run out of pastry. Fold the last flap of pastry underneath the triangular-shaped food parcel. Do the same with the other sheets of pastry. Work swiftly and boldly and you'll soon get the hang of it.

4 Brush or spray the Samosas with the remaining oil and place on the prepared baking tray. Bake on the top shelf of the preheated oven for about 25 minutes, or until the Samosas are golden brown and crispy.

Smoked salmon in bread parcel rolls
Makes 18

Smoked salmon is a good source of omega-3, which has beneficial effects on heart health.

Serve two or three of these per person as a starter with slices of cucumber and tomato to garnish.

Ingredients

6 thin slices from a large wholemeal loaf, crusts removed

40 g (1½ oz) unsaturated margarine

115 g (4 oz) smoked salmon, thinly sliced

juice of 1 lemon

2 tbsp fresh parsley, chopped

freshly ground black pepper

Nutritional analysis

Per parcel, 44 kcals (185 kJ), 2 g fat, of which saturated fat negligible, 181 mg sodium.

Method

1 Thinly spread the margarine on to each slice of bread.

2 Place some smoked salmon on each slice of bread, season and sprinkle with lemon juice and chopped parsley. Then roll each slice up lengthways. Wrap the parcels in foil, then place in the fridge for half an hour. Cut each parcel into 3 slices before serving.

Sardine paté
Serves 2–4

You can make lots of heart-friendly dishes using oily fish and this recipe (from *How to Keep Your Cholesterol in Check*) uses sardines to provide a tasty starter or lunchtime snack. Serve it with toast or crispbread.

Ingredients

1 tin sardines, drained	1 tsp lemon juice
2 tsp low-fat fromage frais, or	freshly ground black pepper
to taste	watercress, to garnish

Nutritional analysis

For 2 servings, per serving, 108 kcals (454 kJ), 6 g fat, of which 1 g saturated, 208 mg sodium.
For 4 servings, per serving, 54 kcals (227 kJ), 3 g fat, of which 1 g saturated, 104 mg sodium.

Method

1 Mix together the sardines and fromage frais.
2 Add the lemon juice and season to taste with black pepper.
3 Garnish with the watercress.

Variation

Try using other oily fish, such as smoked mackerel. This paté recipe using tuna also makes an excellent filling for a baked potato.

Soups

Gazpacho
Serves 6

This traditional Spanish soup, served chilled, is a wonderful liquid salad, full of heart-healthy ingredients. It makes an excellent starter for a summer barbecue.

To make skinning the tomatoes a doddle, place the tomatoes in a suitable bowl and soak them in boiling water for a couple of minutes. Then, just peel the skin off with your thumb.

Ingredients

700 g (1½ lbs) firm, ripe tomatoes, skinned, deseeded and roughly chopped
½ cucumber, peeled and roughly chopped
1 large green pepper, deseeded and roughly chopped
2 garlic cloves, roughly chopped

1½ tbsp red or white wine vinegar
1 tbsp olive oil
115 g (4 oz) breadcrumbs
½ tsp sugar
freshly ground black pepper
275–425 ml (½–¾ pint) cold water
1 red onion, sliced, to garnish

Nutritional analysis

Per serving, 117 kcals (491 kJ), 3 g fat, of which saturated fat negligible, 160 mg sodium.

Method

1 Place all the ingredients – reserving a little of the tomato, cucumber and green pepper, as well as the onion slices – in a food processor with a little water. Add black pepper to taste then process the mixture until it has a smooth consistency.
2 Add sufficient extra water to make into a soup. How thick you make the soup is a matter of choice, but you shouldn't need more than 275–425 ml (½–¾ pint) of water in total – less if you prefer a thick soup.
3 Taste and add more black pepper and a little more sugar if required.

4 Pour the soup into a large bowl, cover with clingfilm and place in the fridge. Chill for a couple of hours before serving. As an accompaniment, provide a 'help yourself' bowl of the reserved vegetable garnish ingredients and some cold croûtons (see recipe for Garlic toasties earlier on page 54).

Leek and potato soup
Serves 4

An old favourite that is good for you. Leeks are a member of the onion family and, as a top antioxidant provider, help to keep our hearts healthy.

Ingredients

2 tsp olive oil
1 medium onion, finely chopped
1 large potato, peeled and diced
2 large leeks, trimmed top and bottom and chopped (as described on page 104)
freshly ground black pepper

570 ml (1 pint) Vegetable stock (see pages 104–5) or use vegetable stock cubes or granules diluted as advised on page 104
200 ml ($\frac{1}{3}$ pint) soya or semi-skimmed milk
1 tbsp fresh parsley or chives, chopped, to garnish

Nutritional analysis
Per serving 106 kcals (445 kJ), 2 g fat, of which saturated fat negligible, 330 mg of sodium.

Method
1 Heat the oil in a flameproof casserole dish or large saucepan. Add the onion and potato and cook over a gentle heat for 3 minutes while preparing the leeks.
2 Add the chopped leeks to the dish or pan. Stir, season to taste with black pepper, then cover and leave to sweat over a very gentle heat for 20 minutes.
3 Add the stock and milk and bring to the boil, then allow to simmer gently for 20 minutes or until the vegetables have cooked.
4 Place the contents of the dish or pan in a food processor and blend (or push through a sieve) to form a purée. Return to the casserole, check the seasoning, reheat, then serve, garnished with the chopped parsley or chives.

Butternut squash soup
Serves 6

Butternut squash is high in the ACE antioxidant vitamins – beta-carotene (vitamin A) and vitamins C and E. It is a very versatile ingredient in both savoury and sweet dishes. Apart from this delicious soup, try roasting it with a little olive oil and thyme, for example, or adding to apple with cinnamon and ginger. To roast, bake it at about 200°C (400°F/gas mark 6) for 40 minutes, turning halfway. With pumpkin (see *Variation* on page 65), you can roast it in slices, cut like melon wedges.

Ingredients

2 tsp vegetable oil
1 medium onion, peeled and finely chopped
1 tsp curry powder
1 butternut squash (about 700 g/1½ lbs), peeled and cut in half, seeds scooped out, flesh cut into chunks
1 large potato, peeled and roughly chopped
1 eating apple, peeled, cored and chopped

few pinches freshly ground nutmeg
1.2 litres (2 pints) Vegetable stock (page 104) or use vegetable stock cubes or granules diluted as advised on page 104
freshly ground black pepper
few sprigs fresh parsley, chopped, to garnish

Nutritional analysis
Per serving, 106 kcals (445 kJ), 2 g fat, of which less than 1 g saturated, 402 mg sodium.

Method
1 Warm the oil in a flameproof casserole dish. Add the onion, then cover and cook over a gentle heat for 5–6 minutes, until softened.
2 Stir in the curry powder and add the chunks of butternut squash together with the potato, apple and nutmeg. Mix together, cover and allow to sweat over a very low heat for 10 minutes, stirring occasionally. Add all but 150 ml (¼ pint) of the stock and bring to the boil.
3 Cover and simmer for about 20 minutes, until the vegetables are tender. Allow to cool slightly, then, using a straining spoon, transfer the vegetables to a food processor or liquidizer. It's nice to leave some texture in the soup, so blend very briefly (about

1 second only) with the reserved stock. Return to the dish, season to taste with pepper and reheat gently. Garnish with the parsley. Serve with warm rolls or croûtons.

Variation
Pumpkin soup
If you're buying a pumpkin at Hallowe'en, you could try substituting a 1-kg ($2\frac{1}{4}$-lb) pumpkin for the butternut squash – this should produce about 500 g (1 lb 2 oz) flesh (the same as the butternut squash). Pumpkin seeds can also be eaten. They are an excellent source of omega-3 and may be of help in managing prostate problems.

Apple and celery soup
Serves 4

Ingredients

2 tsp olive oil
1 head of celery (about 225 g/ 8 oz), trimmed top and bottom, washed and stalks chopped
1 medium onion, finely chopped
2 juicy eating apples, peeled, sliced and cored (Royal Gala apples blend in nicely)
570 ml (1 pint) Vegetable stock (see page 104) or use

vegetable stock cubes or granules diluted as advised on page 104
200 ml ($\frac{1}{3}$ pint) soya or semi-skimmed milk
1 tbsp dry sherry
1 bay leaf
freshly ground black pepper
few sprigs fresh mint or parsley, chopped, to garnish

Nutritional analysis
Per serving, 80 kcals (336 kJ), 3 g fat, of which saturated fat negligible, 350 mg sodium.

Method
1 Gently heat the oil in a flameproof casserole or large saucepan and add the celery and onion. Cover and cook over a low heat for about 10 minutes, or until soft, stirring from time to time to prevent burning.

2 Add the apples and cook for a further 5 minutes.

3 Add the stock, milk, sherry and bay leaf and season to taste with black pepper. Bring to the boil, then simmer gently with the lid on for about 1 hour, or until the vegetables are tender. Remove the bay leaf.

4 Place the rest of the contents in a food processor (or push them through a sieve) and blend into a purée. Then return the purée to the casserole, check the seasoning, reheat gently and serve, topped with the chopped mint or parsley.

Variation
Try stirring in a teaspoon of curry powder at step 2 to add some aromatic Asian flair.

For a tasty Lentil and tomato soup, see under 'Meals in under 30 minutes' (page 155) and for a Thick vegetable soup see page 105.

Salads, sauces, chutneys, marmalade and jam

Salsa Mexicana (Wallman style)
Serves 4

This is a spicy side dish that goes well with Mexican or Indian food. Try it with the Beef or Quorn fajitas (pages 86–7). It can also provide a tasty filling on its own for pitta bread.

Ingredients

5 ripe tomatoes, roughly chopped

1 small red onion, finely chopped

1–2 jalapeños or red chillies, finely chopped (remove seeds if you prefer the salsa less hot)

2 garlic cloves, peeled and crushed

10 ml (2 tsp) cider or white wine vinegar

$\frac{1}{2}$ tsp sugar

2–3 sprigs fresh coriander, roughly chopped

Nutritional information
Per serving, 30 kcals (126 kJ), negligible fat, 11 mg sodium.

Method
1 Place all the ingredients in a bowl and mix together by hand (not in a blender).

Couscous salad
Serves 4

A lovely side salad or excellent accompaniment to barbecue meals.

Ingredients

225 g (8 oz) couscous
275 ml (10 fl oz) boiling water
4 tomatoes, diced
5 spring onions, sliced
½ cucumber, diced
juice of 1 lemon

2 tsp olive oil
2 tsp balsamic vinegar
few sprigs fresh mint, finely
  chopped
few sprigs fresh parsley,
  chopped

Nutritional analysis
Per serving, 170 kcals (714 kJ), 2 g fat, of which saturated fat negligible, 12 mg sodium.

Method
1 Put the couscous into a suitable serving bowl and add the boiling water. Stir once, then cover and leave to stand for 10 minutes or until the couscous has soaked up all the water.
2 Add the tomatoes, spring onions and cucumber to the couscous. Then mix in the lemon juice, olive oil and balsamic vinegar.
3 Finally, stir in the mint and parsley.

French dressing
Serves 2

An easy, delicious dressing for salads.

Ingredients

2 tbsp olive oil
1 tbsp cider or white wine
  vinegar
pinch freshly ground black
  pepper

½ tsp mustard
2 tbsp chopped fresh herbs or
  pinch dry mixed herbs

Nutritional analysis
Per 25-ml (1-fl oz) serving, 42 kcals (176 kJ) – a typical recipe for French dressing provides around 124 kcals (520 kJ).

Method
1 Put all the ingredients in a small jar or bottle and, with the lid screwed on tightly, shake them all together vigorously, maracas-style.

Pear and apple chutney
Makes approximately 1.8–2.3 kg (4–5 lbs)

Full of antioxidants and flavonoids, this home-made chutney spices up cold meat, salads and sandwiches. The recipe uses turmeric, which should be used with care since it can stain – but it may also sustain! One of its constituents is curcumin and there is some evidence to suggest that this may help to sustain good health by reducing the risk of developing a variety of cancers. The recipe offers a blend of pears and apples. Conference pears and Cox or Worcester apples seem to go together particularly well, but you can experiment with different varieties – and with other fruits and vegetables – to suit your own taste. Just gather together 2 kg (4½ lbs) of fruit (weighed before peeling). You can use windfalls, but remember to cut out the bruised parts before weighing the fruit. The chutney is best left for two to three months to mature before using.

Ingredients
3–4 large, mild onions (about 700 g/1½ lbs

1 kg (2¼ lbs) pears, peeled, cored and roughly chopped

1 kg (2¼ lbs) apples, peeled, cored and roughly chopped

170 g (6 oz) sultanas

1 garlic clove

25 g (1 oz) pickling spice, tied in a piece of muslin or gauze

285 g (10 oz) soft dark brown sugar

500 ml (just under 1 pint) cider or white wine vinegar

1 heaped tbsp cornflour

1–2 tbsp water, if required at Step 2

1 tsp turmeric

1–2 tbsp cold water for mixing

Nutritional analysis
Per 450-g (1-lb) jar, 631 kcals (2650 kJ), 1 g fat, of which saturated fat negligible, 54 mg sodium.

Method
1 Crush the garlic, finely chop the onions and place in a preserving pan, together with the apples, pears and sultanas. Add the pickling spice and vinegar.
2 Bring to the boil, then allow to simmer very gently over a low heat. Stir occasionally to make sure that the mixture does not burn

and to check the liquid level. If it gets too dry, add 1–2 tablespoons of water. Allow the mixture to cook down until it forms a thick purée and the onion is soft and tender. This can take an hour or more.

3 Add the sugar and stir until dissolved. Bring back to the boil and simmer for 5 minutes.

4 Remove the pickling spice and mix the cornflour and turmeric together with a little cold water to form a smooth paste. Stir this into the mixture and bring it back to the boil briefly, stirring until it has thickened. Turmeric is a mild spice but has a strong pigment that gives added colour to food such as curry, rice and chutney. Take care handling it as it can stain quite badly.

5 Sterilize the jars by preheating them in a 180°C (350°F/gas mark 4) oven for 5 minutes. Pour the hot chutney immediately into the warm jars and cover in the usual way. Leave to cook, then store in a cool place.

Mango chutney
Makes 1.4–1.8 kg (3–4 lbs)

A traditional accompaniment to curries, this recipe produces a chutney with a lovely fresh, fruity taste. Try it with the Curry on pages 96–7 or the Cheat's curry recipe on page 164.

The chutney is best left for a week or two before using as this allows the flavours to blend.

Ingredients

4 large mangoes, just starting to ripen but not too soft, each about 500–600 g (1 lb 2 oz–1 lb 6 oz)
1 garlic clove, crushed
2 tsp ground coriander
2 tsp ground ginger
275 ml ($\frac{1}{2}$ pint) cider vinegar
115 g (4 oz) soft dark brown sugar

Nutritional analysis
Per 450-g (1-lb) jar, 200 kcals (840 kJ), of which fat negligible, 16 mg sodium.

Method

1 Wash the mangoes, then slice them lengthways, on either side of the stone, to leave 3 pieces. Clean the flesh from the piece containing the stone as much as possible, then enjoy nibbling the rest off as the chef's perk! Cut the mango flesh into small chunks, then take the other two pieces and slice them thinly lengthwise without removing the skin. Cut the slices into small pieces about 2.5 cm (1 in) long. Do the same for each mango.

2 Place the mango chunks in a large saucepan with the rest of the ingredients, apart from the sugar. Mix together well. Bring to the boil, cutting any large pieces of skin you find in the mixture with kitchen scissors. Bring to the boil and simmer gently for about 45 minutes, or until the skin is soft and the mixture forms a thick, chutney-like purée. The mixture should thicken on its own without the need to add cornflour. Stir occasionally to prevent burning.

3 Add the sugar and stir until it has dissolved. Bring back to the boil and simmer for about 10 minutes, stirring frequently.

4 Sterilize the jars by preheating them in a 180°C (350°F/gas mark 4) oven for 5 minutes. Pour the hot chutney immediately into the warm jars and cover in the usual. way. Leave them to cool, then store in a cool place.

Grapefruit and lemon marmalade
Makes about 2.8 kg (6 lbs)

Like oranges, grapefruits and lemons are low in fat and calories. These fruits are also full of cholesterol-lowering pectin, and vitamin C. So enjoy your marmalade as a special morning treat, knowing that it is doing you good!

Note that if you want to make less marmalade, just reduce the ingredients in proportion. For example, you can make a couple of small jars (about 675 g/1½ lbs) by using 1 grapefruit and 1 lemon with a quarter of the water and sugar in a large saucepan. The setting point will be reached in about half the time.

Ingredients

3–4 large grapefruit, about
1.4 kg (3 lbs) total weight
4 medium unwaxed lemons,
about 450–550 g (1–1¼ lbs)
total weight

1.7 litres (3 pints) water
1.4 kg (3 lbs) sugar

Nutritional analysis

For Grapefruit and lemon marmalade, per 450-g (1-lb) jar, 1005 kcals (4221 kJ), negligible fat, 22 mg sodium. For Orange and lemon marmalade, 690 kcals (2898 kJ), of which fat negligible, 19 mg sodium. 1 level tsp marmalade has about 4 g added sugar.

Method

1 Wash the fruit. Peel off the grapefruit and lemon zest – zest only, as little pith as possible – very thinly using a potato peeler or very sharp knife. Then, finely slice the cut peel with scissors. You'll find you can cut through several pieces at once.
2 Next, peel off the pith from the fruit and set it aside. Chop up the flesh roughly, reserving the pips, and place it in a preserving pan with the juice that has been produced by chopping and the water.
3 Tie the reserved pith and pips from the fruit in a large piece of muslin, attach it to the pan with string and dangle it in the water with the fruit. Bring to the boil and simmer gently for 1 to 1½ hours, or until the contents of the pan have reduced by half and the peel is very soft.
4 Remove the muslin bag, squeezing it out over the pan (tongs are useful for this).
5 Add the sugar and bring back to the boil, stirring all the time. Then, boil rapidly until the setting point is reached (about 10 minutes), stirring frequently. To check for setting, take a spoonful of the marmalade, place it on a saucer and leave in the fridge for about 5 minutes. (Don't forget to take the pan off the heat while you are checking the marmalade.) The marmalade is set if the surface forms wrinkles when you draw your finger across it. If it isn't ready, boil it for a few moments more.
6 Allow to cool for about 10 minutes before putting the marmalade into warm jars in the usual way.

Variation
Orange and lemon marmalade
You can make this delicious variation by substituting the same weight of ordinary large oranges for the grapefruit and reducing the sugar content by one-third. This makes three to four 450-g (1-lb) jars of marmalade.

Plum jam
Makes approximately 2.25 kg (5 lbs)

Plums (and damsons) are a good source of vitamin E – one of the antioxidants that is important in the prevention of heart disease. Another plus is that plums (and damsons) have a low glycaemic index.

Ingredients
1.4 kg (3 lbs) plums
425 ml ($\frac{3}{4}$ pint) water
1 kg ($2\frac{1}{4}$ lbs) sugar

Nutritional analysis
Per 450-g (1-lb) jar, 889 kcals (3734 kJ), of which saturated fat negligible, 16 mg sodium. 1 level tsp jam has about 4 g added sugar.

Method
1 Wash the plums, cut them in half and take out the stones.
2 Place the fruit and water in a preserving pan. Bring to the boil and simmer for about 45 minutes, or until the fruit is very soft, stirring occasionally.
3 Add the sugar and stir until it has dissolved. Then, bring the contents of the pan to a full, rolling boil until the setting point is reached (it sets quite quickly, often within 2 to 3 minutes). Check as described in step 5 on page 73, removing the pan from the heat while you do so.
4 Transfer to warmed jars.

Mincemeat
Makes approximately 900 g (2 lbs)

Medieval mincemeat did actually contain meat of various kinds, chopped up and mixed with suet and fruit and served as a starter. Over time, the meat was gradually left out in favour of fruits, spices and brandy, and it is the sweet mincemeat that has found its way into the mince pies we enjoy today.

Traditionally, mincemeat uses suet, which is especially high in saturated fat. However, as this recipe shows, you don't need to use *any* added fat.

Try this as the filling for your Christmas mince pies or spooned into the centres of baked apples. The mincemeat is better if it is left to mature for a few weeks before using.

Ingredients
250 g (9 oz) ready-to-eat dried apricots, cut into raisin-sized pieces
115 g (4 oz) glacé cherries, cut into eighths
225g (8 oz) raisins
225 g (8 oz) sultanas
225 g (8 oz) currants
100 g ($3\frac{1}{2}$ oz) candied peel, chopped
juice and grated rind of 2 lemons
225 g (8 oz) cooking apples, peeled, cored and grated
200 g (7 oz) soft dark brown sugar
2 tsp mixed spice
150 ml ($\frac{1}{4}$ pint) brandy

Nutritional analysis
Per 450-g (1-lb) jar, 1944 kcals (8164 kJ), 3 g fat, of which saturated fat negligible, 313 mg sodium. Per Mince pie (page 144–5), 86 kcals (361 kJ), negligible fat, negligible saturated fat, 14 mg sodium.

Method
1 Place all the ingredients – apart from the brandy – in a large bowl and mix together well.
2 Cover the bowl with clingfilm and allow the flavours to blend together for 48 hours, if possible, in a cool place. Stir the mixture occasionally.
3 Finally, add the brandy a little at a time and stir the mixture well.
4 Transfer to warmed jars.

Main courses – fish, meat and vegetarian dishes

Fish

Fish provide an excellent source of nutrients, including protein. In fact, one large portion of fish can contain up to half our daily protein requirements – white fish, such as cod, haddock or plaice, rival meat in this respect. Most fish also contain iodine, needed by the thyroid gland, and vitamin B12, which is essential to the smooth functioning of the nervous system. Fish also contain iron in a form that the body can easily absorb.

Oily fish, such as mackerel, herring, sardine, trout, salmon and tuna, have specific benefits for our circulatory systems, helping us to avoid strokes and heart disease. They are a good source of vitamins A, B12 and D, and fish oil is rich in the heart-healthy omega-3 family of fatty acids (apart from tinned tuna as most of the omega-3 content is removed during the cooking process that precedes canning). Omega-3 fatty acids help to lower triglyceride levels, prevent irregularities in the heart's rhythm and stop the blood from getting too sticky. The omega-3 in oily fish may also help to lower blood pressure and increase life expectancy, even for people with existing heart disease. There is also some indication that eating omega-3-rich foods as part of a Mediterranean diet might play a part in protecting from certain forms of cancer, reduce joint pain and inflammation in conditions such as rheumatoid arthritis, and help to prevent the deterioration in mental functioning among older age groups.

The only downside with fish, especially oily fish, is that they are at risk of being contaminated by toxins in our rivers and seas and some oily fish have been found to contain traces of mercury. The advice from most dietitians is that the heart health benefits of eating oily fish still far outweigh any slight risk of mercury poisoning. However, because mercury can cause damage to the nervous system of foetuses and young children, some groups of people, such as children under 16, women who are pregnant or planning a pregnancy or mothers who are breastfeeding, are advised to limit their intake of certain fish. These are the fish that have a longer lifespan than other fish and are, therefore, likely to have built up higher concentrations of mercury. It is therefore suggested that these groups limit their intake of tuna to two medium-sized cans or one fresh tuna steak per week and that they avoid fish such as marlin, swordfish and shark altogether.

For most other people, the current recommendation is that eating two portions of fish a week (one oily) is a safe and healthy option. This is the amount currently advised by the Food Standards Agency, but, for people with heart disease, the British Dietetic Association recommends an intake of two to three portions of oily fish every week, where a portion is 100 g (4 oz). For those who cannot eat fish, a concentrated fish oil supplement can be taken that provides 1 g omega-3 fats daily. A pure supplement is recommended, rather than those mixed with other vitamins.

Fish can be cooked in all sorts of ways – grilling, poaching and baking are especially healthy approaches.

Grilling

Grilling gives fish a lovely crisp finish. It works best with subtly flavoured flat fish, such as plaice or sole, but be careful not to let the flesh dry out. This method is also excellent for oily fish, which are less likely to dry out anyway.

If you have time, marinate the fish with a little olive oil and lemon juice to ensure that it stays moist and to add flavour. Otherwise, brush or spray with a little unsaturated fat before cooking. If you're cooking whole fish, slash the skin a few times at the thickest part to let the heat penetrate.

To cook, preheat the grill to a medium high heat for 5 minutes. Place the fish on a piece of foil quite near the heat. When the outside starts to look slightly crisp and golden, turn to cook the other side. Don't be tempted to turn the fish more than once. It should take eight to ten minutes to cook.

Poaching

This is probably the best way to enjoy the pure natural flavours of fresh fish, especially if you plan to eat it cold. The fish can be poached, for example, in milk or water, seasoned with wine, cider or stock.

This method works well with white fish and shellfish. Salmon and trout also poach beautifully, but the method doesn't work so well with other oily fish.

For a tasty stock, make a *court bouillon*. All you need to do is add a sliced onion, a sliced carrot, a bay leaf, a few sprigs of thyme and

5 tablespoons of cider vinegar to 570 ml (1 pint) of water in a saucepan, simmer the mixture gently, covered, for 30 minutes, then cool and strain.

Now you're ready to poach your fish. The gentlest way to poach is to add the fish to the cold *court bouillon* or your preferred stock. Bring it to a gentle simmer, but never allow the water to boil as the flavour of the fish will escape into the water and the flesh will break down. Drain and allow to cool before serving.

As to cooking times, you'll find that thin fish will be cooked just as the stock starts to simmer, but chunks of fish should be allowed to simmer for around 5 minutes and larger pieces for 15 to 20 minutes.

Roasting in parcels

Cut a piece of greaseproof paper roughly four times the size of the fish. Place the fish on the paper with a few lemon wedges and seasoning. Add some freshly sliced vegetables, herbs and a splash of wine. Scrunch the paper at the edges and fold them in to seal.

For a small whole fish or fillets or steaks, bake in a preheated 200°C (400°F/gas mark 5) oven for 15 to 20 minutes. For a large whole fish, set the temperature to 180°C (350°F/gas mark 4) and bake for 30 to 40 minutes. Serve the fish in its parcel.

Paté

Fish also makes excellent paté and we have included a tasty recipe for Sardine (or smoked mackerel) paté on page 61. Another fish recipe that makes a lovely starter is Smoked salmon in bread parcel rolls (page 60).

What to look for when buying fresh fish

Whole fish

The eyes should be bright and the flesh shiny and moist, with a firm appearance and bright colour.

Fresh fillets

These should be neatly trimmed and have a nice bright colour and plump, glossy flesh with no signs of dryness or breaking up.

Smoked fish

All smoked fish should have a lovely glossy appearance and a fresh smoky aroma.

Salmon or tuna steak with tomato, basil and red wine sauce
Serves 4

Fish such as salmon and tuna are rich in omega-3 fatty acids, which help to reduce blood stickiness and keep triglyceride levels low. They also protect the heart from arrhythmias.

If you use the grilling method given, the whole meal can be ready in less than half an hour, so you could also count this recipe as belonging in the 'Meals in under 30 minutes' section! It is delicious served with new potatoes and French beans.

Try this recipe when you have a barbecue. Simply follow the instructions for grilling, but dispense with the foil and place the fish directly on the barbecue griddle.

Ingredients

4 x 115-g (4-oz) salmon or
  tuna steaks

juice of 1 lemon
freshly ground black pepper

For the sauce

1 medium onion, finely
  chopped
1 medium red pepper,
  deseeded and diced
2 tsp extra virgin olive oil
1 garlic clove, crushed or
  finely chopped

2 large tomatoes, chopped
1 tsp fresh basil, chopped
1 tbsp tomato ketchup
1 tbsp red wine

Nutritional analysis
Per serving, 220 kcals (924 kJ), 10 g fat, of which 2 g saturated, 137 mg sodium.

Method
1 Wash the fish and place on cooking foil. Sprinkle half the lemon juice over one side of the steaks and season to taste with pepper. Allow to marinate for 10 minutes. Turn the steaks over and marinate the other side for the same length of time.
2 While the steaks are marinating, prepare the sauce and preheat the oven to 170°C (325°F/gas mark 3) if you are oven baking the fish. Cook the onion and red pepper in a covered saucepan with the oil

over a low heat for about 5–6 minutes, or until the onion and pepper are soft.

3 Add the garlic, tomatoes and basil, together with the ketchup and red wine. Season to taste with pepper. Cook over a gentle heat for about 10 minutes. Take off the heat and allow to stand until the fish is nearly cooked, then reheat.

4 *To grill:* place the steaks on the foil under a medium heat and grill for about 5 minutes each side. Reheat the sauce and spoon over the fish steaks before serving.

To oven bake: spoon the sauce over the steaks and make the foil into a parcel. Bake in the preheated oven for 30 minutes.

Rock-a-Nore fish crumble
Serves 4

Hastings boasts one of the largest fleets of beach-launched fishing craft in the UK. This recipe is named after Rock-a-Nore – the area of the town that houses the local fish market, where freshly caught fish is sold daily.

Ingredients
For the crumble
50 g (2 oz) rolled oats
50 g (2 oz) wholemeal
 breadcrumbs

50 g (2 oz) low-fat (16 per
 cent) cheese, grated
cayenne pepper

For the filling
1 tbsp olive oil
2 shallots,
 finely chopped
225 g (8 oz) broccoli,
 prepared as described
 in step 3 overleaf
115 g (4 oz) button
 mushrooms, sliced
25 g (1 oz) wholemeal
 flour
275 ml ($\frac{1}{2}$ pint)
 semi-skimmed
 or soya milk

115 g (4 oz) frozen
 sweetcorn
 or equivalent
 drained weight
 tinned sweetcorn
freshly ground black
 pepper
450 g (1 lb) white fish
 fillets, skinned
2 tomatoes,
 sliced

Nutritional analysis
Per serving, 323 kcals (1357 kJ), 9 g fat, of which 3 g saturated,
258 mg sodium.

Method
1 Preheat the oven to 200°C (400°F/gas mark 6) and prepare the
  crumble by mixing together the ingredients in a bowl and adding
  cayenne pepper to taste.
2 Next, make the filling. Heat the oil in a frying pan and gently
  sauté the shallots for 5 minutes.
3 Chop the broccoli stalks into thin slices, reserving the florets. Add
  the stalks to the pan, along with the mushrooms. Fry over a gentle
  heat for about 5 minutes and then stir in the flour, followed by
  the milk, broccoli florets and sweetcorn. Simmer for a further
  5 minutes, stirring continuously in order to mix ingredients and
  prevent sticking. Season to taste with black pepper.
4 Put the fish into a medium-sized casserole or pie dish and pour the
  filling mixture over it. Spread the ingredients over the fish, then
  spoon the crumble mixture over the top and level it off.
5 Bake in the preheated oven for 35–40 minutes or until the broccoli
  has cooked, the filling is bubbling nicely and the top has browned
  lightly.
6 Garnish with the tomato slices. Serve piping hot with boiled or
  baked potatoes, other vegetables of your choice and a dash of
  tomato ketchup.

Kedgeree
Serves 4

This recipe uses basmati rice which is the lowest on the glycaemic
index of any of the varieties of rice. Keeping low on this index helps
to keep weight under control, lowers glucose concentrations and
increases levels of HDL cholesterol.

If you want to make the Kedgeree resemble the traditional Indian
kichri a little more closely, just add half a teaspoon of turmeric to the
milk at step 4 so that the rice takes on a yellowish tinge.

A slice of bread goes nicely with this dish, as does tomato ketchup
or Mango chutney (pages 70–1). It also freezes well and can be
reheated in the microwave.

Ingredients

225 g (8 oz) haddock or any
  other white fish
225 g (8 oz) smoked haddock
425 ml ($\frac{3}{4}$ pint) semi-skimmed
  or soya milk
2 hard-boiled eggs, chopped
1 tsp olive oil
2 spring onions, chopped

225 g (8 oz) basmati rice
2 tsp curry paste
115 g (4 oz) frozen peas,
  cooked
freshly ground black pepper
sliced tomatoes, chopped fresh
  parsley and lemon wedges
  to garnish

Nutritional analysis

Per serving, 414 kcals (1739 kJ), 7 g fat, of which 2 g saturated,
613 mg sodium.

Method

1 Place the fish in a deep frying pan and cover with the milk. Poach
  gently until just cooked (about 10–15 minutes). Prepare the hard-
  boiled eggs while the fish is cooking.
2 Strain off the milk into a jug and transfer the fish to a cutting
  board. Flake the fish, detaching flesh from the skin with a fork.
  Remove any stray bones and wrap in foil to keep it warm.
3 Rinse out the pan, add the oil and heat gently. Add the onions and
  cook over a low heat until tender. Stir in the curry paste and cook
  for a further minute.
4 Stir the rice into the mixture and then pour in the reserved milk.
  Stir gently to mix the contents, heat until it starts to simmer, then
  cover with a lid and leave to cook for about 15 minutes. About 5
  minutes before the rice is ready, cook the frozen peas separately.
6 Remove the frying pan from the heat and fork in the fish, hard-
  boiled eggs and peas. Return to the heat and cook gently for about
  5 more minutes, until the mixture is nice and hot. Add a little
  more milk if necessary. Add pepper to taste, turn out into a
  warmed serving bowl and garnish with the tomato slices, chopped
  parsley and lemon wedges.

Meat and vegetarian

We have offered a vegetarian alternative to all the meat dishes
included, so just choose a recipe you'd like to try and the vegetarian
version is there with it, too.

Meat and vegetables are both rich in nutrients. We have described the powerful antioxidant benefits of vegetables in Chapter 3 and later in the Recipes section under 'Vegetables and fruit'. Meat does not provide these antioxidant benefits directly, but it does provide zinc in a form that the body finds easy to absorb and, by assisting enzymes that attack them, zinc helps in the fight against free radicals. So, indirectly, meat also has a role to play in keeping free radicals at bay. It also contains other nutrients that help our bodies to function efficiently. For example, it provides a good source of iron and, like fish, provides it in a form that our bodies can readily absorb. This contrasts with the iron found in other foods, such as eggs, dark green leafy vegetables, beans and cereals. In these foods the iron, while just as valuable, is less easily absorbed by our bodies. We can, though, improve iron absorption from these sources by ensuring a good intake of vitamin C (from citrus fruits or juices, for example) – advice that is especially important for vegetarians.

To make red blood cells, we need a number of ingredients – especially iron, vitamin B12 and folic acid. A deficiency in one or more of these will result in anaemia, which is when the body doesn't produce enough red blood cells. Meat is also a good source of protein and it is especially rich in the B vitamins, including vitamin B12. We only require minute quantities of vitamin B12 (also obtained from white fish, yeast extract, eggs, milk and fortified cereals), but it is important for cell formation and growth and for the nourishment of the nervous system. If you are a vegan and do not eat any animal foods (meat, fish, eggs or dairy foods) or animal-derived ingredients, you will need to make sure that you obtain this vitamin from another source, such as supplements or fortified foods. For most other people, a balanced diet will provide an adequate supply.

The main drawback with meat from the heart health point of view is that it can contain large amounts of saturated fat of the type that raises the levels of the less desirable LDL cholesterol in our blood. So, you need to be aware of the saturated fat content of various meats, just as you need to be aware of the fat content of other foods. First of all, though, we need to dispel one myth – that you need to cut out red meat to follow a cholesterol-lowering diet. This is simply wrong. Although *fatty* cuts of red meat are generally high in saturates, *lean* cuts are relatively low. For example, lean beef can contain less than 5 per cent fat, of which only 2 per cent is saturated. Red meat will contain some dietary cholesterol, but this isn't usually a problem for most people and the downside is counterbalanced by the fact that meat also contains quite substantial amounts of cholesterol-lowering monounsaturated and polyunsaturated fat, together with some beneficial omega-3 fatty acids. So, if you like a bit of lean beef, go ahead and have it.

White meats, such as turkey and chicken, generally have a low saturated fat content. Lean ham, too, is low in fat. You need to check on the fat content of other meats, such as lamb and pork, but, if you are careful and select meat from which the fat has been trimmed off, you can often find pork with only about 4 per cent fat and lamb that has around 8 per cent fat. So, hunt around for low-fat cuts.

Bacon, sausages, meat pies and mince all tend to be on the high-fat, high-saturates side – you need to check the food label for such items. Whatever you choose, though, you can help yourselves by grilling rather than frying. This way, you will allow much of the fat to escape before you eat the meat. Indeed, we suggest that you *do* allow it to escape rather than capture it again in the form of a fatty gravy. As far as heart health is concerned, the best option is to make some gravy from suitable low-fat gravy granules, using the water from cooking the vegetables rather than the juices and fat from cooking the meat. Alternatively, it is possible to buy special gravy jugs that separate off the fat for you.

As far as vegetables are concerned, there are no health drawbacks and it is relatively easy to produce lovely vegetables from your own garden, allotment or from tubs on your balcony or patio. With a small amount of effort and little expense, you can have a ready supply of nutritious – and organic – cooking ingredients. It's surprising how many vegetables you can grow in a relatively small space. Even in gardens predominantly filled with flowers and shrubs, there's always space for a few lettuces, some runner beans by the fence or a pot of cherry tomatoes on the patio.

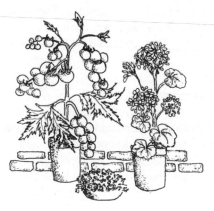

Some suggestions for a summer barbecue

- The Garlic toasties (page 54) make an excellent starter. Just place the bread directly on to the griddle. Watch them closely so they don't burn because they're ready in a flash.
- Try the Salmon or tuna steak with tomato, basil and red wine sauce recipe (pages 78–9), using the foil-wrapped method.
- Vegetarian options include vegetarian sausages and vegeburgers or try mini Quorn fillets with different flavourings, such as tikka. These are best cooked with added marinade to prevent them drying out. You could use the marinade recipe given below for basting vegetables. You can also cut up meat or Quorn fillets and thread on to skewers with your favourite chopped vegetables.
- For vegetables on a skewer, you could have courgette in 0.5-cm ($\frac{1}{4}$-in) thick slices, with chunks of red, green or yellow peppers, whole shallots and whole button mushrooms or, indeed, anything you fancy that will cook quickly. The vegetables mentioned only take 5 or 6 minutes to cook.
- Baste the vegetables with a marinade of the juice of 1 lemon, 1 teaspoon of honey, 1 tablespoon of olive oil and 1 tablespoon of chopped fresh mint. Serve with a side salad of lettuce and tomato or Couscous salad (pages 67–8).
- Finish off with the deliciously cooling Pear or Strawberry sorbet (pages 121–2).

Safety hints

You may have read that barbecuing meat and fish can produce compounds implicated in the development of some forms of cancer (of the colon and stomach, for example). The American Institute for Cancer Research suggests that we needn't consider barbecues off limits because of this, but should just take care to observe a few simple rules to make them as safe as possible:

- trim the fat off meat
- marinate meats very well before grilling as marinating foods can reduce the dangerous compounds by as much as 92–99 per cent
- keep portions small and precook meats and fish to reduce the grilling time
- try to avoid flare-ups from drips by covering the grill with punctured foil or wrapping the meat or fish in foil, for example

- flip the food frequently
- remove any charred or burned parts before eating
- try grilling marinated vegetables on skewers instead of meat (see the suggestions above).

Broccoli and lentil flan
Serves 4

This dish uses a type of flan base made from oats and lentils rather than pastry, with some olive oil and tomato purée to bind everything together. The base is filled with vegetables, covered with a sauce and topped with grated cheese. We have used broccoli in the filling, but you can try different vegetables, such as diced courgettes or sliced mushrooms. A bonus with broccoli is that it is rich in vitamins A, C and E, beta-carotene, riboflavin, calcium and folic acid. An average-sized serving of broccoli contains as much vitamin C as an average-sized orange.

Ingredients
For base
115 g (4 oz) red lentils
1 medium onion, finely
    chopped
1 tsp extra virgin olive oil
1 garlic clove, finely chopped
50 g (2 oz) oats

1 tbsp tomato purée
juice of $\frac{1}{2}$ a lemon
1 tsp dried mixed herbs
dash Tabasco sauce
freshly ground black pepper

For filling
225 g (8 oz) broccoli, divided
    into florets
2 eggs
1 heaped tbsp wholemeal flour
3 tbsp semi-skimmed or soya
    milk

freshly ground black pepper
50 g (2 oz) low-fat (under 16
    per cent) hard cheese, grated
paprika

Nutritional analysis
Per serving, 287 kcals (1205 kJ), 8 g fat, of which 3 g saturated, 159 mg sodium.

Method

1 Preheat the oven to 220°C (425°F/gas mark 7), then put the lentils in a pan and cover with twice their volume of water. Cook for about 10 minutes, until the water has been absorbed and the lentils are quite soft.

2 While the lentils are cooking, place the chopped onion in a large pan with the oil. Cover and cook over a gentle heat for about 4 minutes or until soft. Add the garlic and cook for a further 2 minutes.

3 When the lentils are cooked, drain and transfer to the pan containing the onions and garlic. Mix together.

4 Steam the broccoli florets for about 5 minutes while you finish preparing the base.

5 Stir into the onion and lentil mix the oats, tomato purée, lemon juice and mixed herbs. Add Tabasco sauce and black pepper to taste. The mixture should resemble a very thick paste which will hold together sufficiently to form a base for the filling. Press the mixture into the sides and base of a greased 20-cm (8-in) flan dish. Place the cooked broccoli in the middle.

6 To finish the filling, mix together the eggs, flour and milk. Season with black pepper and pour over the broccoli. Cover with the grated cheese and sprinkle paprika over the top.

7 Bake on the middle shelf of the preheated oven for 30 minutes, or until the filling has set and browned slightly.

Beef or Quorn fajitas
Serves 4

Fajitas traditionally use a tough beef skirt steak, known in Mexico as *arracheras* and *fajitas* in the USA. Vegetarians can enjoy fajitas made using Quorn steaks.

Quorn is a relatively recent discovery. In 1967, new edible fungi (similar to mushrooms and truffles) were found in the UK in a field near Marlow, Buckinghamshire. They were given the name myco-protein. 'Myco' comes from the Greek for fungus and 'protein' draws attention to the fact that the fungus is a good source of protein. Quorn is the brand name of a product that uses this mycoprotein as one of its basic ingredients, so it has a good level of protein as well as being high in fibre and low in fat, providing us with a useful heart-healthy food.

The fajitas are delicious as a light or snack lunch. For a more substantial meal, double up the quantities or use this filling to make the oven-baked enchiladas described in the next recipe.

Ingredients

1 garlic clove, crushed
1 tsp ground cumin
$\frac{1}{2}$ tsp black peppercorns, crushed
juice of 1 lemon
juice of 1 lime
dash of Tabasco sauce

150 g (5 oz) lean beef steak or similar amount of Quorn fillets
1 green pepper
1 shallot
1 tomato
4 large tortillas

Nutritional analysis

Per fajita, 206 kcals (865 kJ), 3 g fat, of which 1 g saturated, 159 mg sodium.

Method

1 To make the marinade, place the garlic, cumin, black peppercorns, lime and lemon juice in a jug. Stir and add a dash of Tabasco sauce to taste.

2 Trim any visible fat off the meat, then cut it or the Quorn into thin strips – enough to provide 2 to 3 for each fajita.

3 Place in a bowl and pour the marinade over them. Make sure that they are well coated and allow the meat or Quorn to marinate in the fridge for at least 1 hour.

4 Deseed the pepper and slice into small strips. Finely chop the shallot and dice the tomato.

5 Wrap the tortillas in foil and warm in the oven, set to 180°C (350°F/gas mark 4), for about 10 to 15 minutes, or wrap in absorbent kitchen paper and heat in the microwave for 1 to 2 minutes, according to instructions.

6 While the tortillas are warming, lightly spray or brush a frying pan or wok with a little unsaturated oil and place over a high heat. Drain the meat or Quorn and add it to the pan, together with the pepper and shallot. Stir-fry the meat for about 5 minutes or Quorn for 10 minutes. Add the tomato 2 minutes before the end of cooking.

7 Turn the fajita mixture into a warmed serving dish. Put some fajita mixture into each tortilla and roll up. Serve with Salsa Mexicana (page 67), crispy lettuce and fromage frais and/or yogurt. Traditionally eaten with the fingers.

Tomato, courgette and chilli enchiladas
Serves 4

Tortillas are a traditional Mexican unleavened bread. In this recipe, they are baked in a sauce to make eight *enchiladas*, which means, literally, 'cooked with some chilli'. They are delicious eaten with a crisp green salad and/or baked potatoes.

Note that you should wash your hands after preparing the chilli because the juice and seeds are very powerful. If you accidentally touch your eyes before you have washed your hands, you can be left with a very painful burning sensation!

Ingredients

1 tbsp extra virgin olive oil
1 large onion, peeled and
  finely chopped
1 red chilli, finely chopped,
  deseeded if you prefer the
  dish less hot
2 garlic cloves, crushed
1 small courgette, sliced
$\frac{1}{2}$ red pepper, deseeded and
  finely chopped

1 level tsp ground cumin
1 level tsp dried oregano
2 x 400-g (14-oz) tins chopped
  tomatoes
1 level tsp sugar
1 tbsp red wine
freshly ground black pepper
50 g (2 oz) low-fat hard
  cheese, grated
8 large tortillas

Nutritional analysis
Per serving, 418 kcals (1756 kJ), 6 g fat, of which 2 g saturated, 474 mg sodium.

Method
1 Preheat the oven to 180°C (350°F/gas mark 4), then place the olive oil in a large saucepan over a low heat. Add the onion and cook with the lid on the pan for about 5 to 6 minutes, or until the onion has softened.
2 Add the chilli, garlic, courgette and pepper and cook gently for another 3 to 4 minutes. Add in the cumin and oregano for the last minute, stirring the mixture to prevent burning.
3 Pour in the tinned tomatoes, add the sugar and red wine, then cook over a low heat for about 20 to 25 minutes, until the mixture makes a thick sauce. Season with pepper to taste.
4 Five minutes before the sauce is ready, wrap the tortillas, stacked

on top of each other, in foil and place in the oven as it is warming up for cooking. Remove when warm – about 10 minutes.

5 Lay the tortillas out flat and spread some of the sauce on each of them, reserving about 2 tablespoons. Roll them up tightly before placing them in an ovenproof dish about 23 cm (9 in) square, making sure that the seam-side lies against the bottom of the dish to stop it opening up during cooking. Spread the reserved sauce on top of the tortillas and sprinkle with the cheese.

6 Bake in the preheated oven for about 30 minutes.

Veggie loaf
Serves 4

The Veggie loaf makes an excellent vegetarian centrepiece for Sunday lunch! Serve it with roast or new potatoes and broccoli or French or runner beans and a little vegetarian gravy. Alternatively, to follow the Indian theme of the curry powder, try it with rice and Mango chutney (pages 70–1).

If you're not keen on curry flavours, though, add a teaspoon of yeast extract at step 3 instead of the curry powder in step 1.

Ingredients

1 tsp olive oil
1 medium onion, finely chopped
1 red pepper, diced
1 red chilli, finely chopped (see page 88) (deseeded for milder flavour, with seeds for more heat)
1 garlic clove, finely chopped
1 tsp curry powder
115 g (4 oz) wholemeal breadcrumbs

25 g (1 oz) chopped mixed nuts
1 medium carrot, grated
115 g (4 oz) mushrooms, chopped into small pieces
freshly ground black pepper
1 egg
1 tbsp tomato purée
handful fresh basil, roughly chopped, to garnish
1 tomato, sliced, to garnish

Nutritional analysis

Per serving, 175 kcals (735 kJ), 7 g fat, of which 1 g saturated, 224 mg sodium (increases to 318 mg if yeast extract used instead of curry powder).

Method

1 Grease a 900-g (2-lb) loaf tin and line it with baking paper, then preheat the oven to 190°C (375°F/gas mark 5). Place the oil in a large pan or flameproof casserole dish with the onion, red pepper, chilli and garlic. Cover and sweat over a low heat for about 10 minutes, until soft, stirring occasionally to prevent sticking. Stir in the curry powder and cook for a further minute. Remove from the heat and set on one side.

2 Place the breadcrumbs, nuts, carrot and mushrooms in a large bowl and mix together. Season to taste with black pepper. Then stir in the cooked vegetables.

3 Mix together the egg and tomato purée in a jug and add to the mixture to help to bind it together. Then, transfer to the prepared loaf tin. Press the mixture down into the tin and level the top. Bake on the middle shelf of the preheated oven for 35 to 40 minutes, or until the top is crisp. Turn out on to a serving plate and garnish with the basil and slices of tomato.

Variations

Vegeburgers

Make 8 vegeburgers by forming the mixture into rounds at step 3. Place on an oiled baking tray and bake at 190°C (375°F/gas mark 5) for about 20–25 minutes.

Stuffed mushrooms

Remove the stalks of 8 large, flat mushrooms. Fill the middle with the mixture, adding the stalks, chopped. Bake in the oven as for the Vegeburgers above.

Stir-fried vegetables with chicken or pork, tofu or Quorn on couscous
Serves 4

Stir-frying is an excellent way of producing low-fat meals, so make double amounts of sweet and sour sauce and freeze the extra. Use any vegetables you fancy.

Ingredients
For the sauce

1 x 432-g (15-oz) (250 g/9 oz drained weight) tin pineapple pieces in natural juice
1 rounded tbsp cornflour
2 tsp honey
2 tsp cider vinegar

2 tsp tomato purée
2 tsp soy sauce
8 tbsp water
2 tbsp dry sherry
$\frac{1}{2}$–1 tsp Tabasco sauce
freshly ground black pepper to taste

For vegetables, meat, tofu or Quorn

2 tsp olive oil
2 shallots, peeled and finely chopped
2 carrots, peeled and cut into matchsticks
1 red pepper, deseeded and sliced
knob fresh root ginger – about 2 tsp when peeled and chopped
1 garlic clove, finely chopped or crushed

225 g (8 oz) chicken breast or pork fillet, thinly sliced, or tofu or Quorn pieces
couscous sufficient for 4 people
115 g (4 oz) mushrooms, sliced
225 g (8 oz) mangetout
handful seedless black grapes, halved
handful peanuts (about 10 g/ $\frac{1}{2}$ oz)

Nutritional analysis
For sauce, per serving, 133 kcals (559 kJ), 0.2 g fat, of which saturated fat negligible, 601 mg sodium (mainly from the soy sauce).

For vegetables, meat, tofu or Quorn (chicken used for analysis), per serving, 150 kcals (630 kJ), 5 g fat, of which 1 g saturated, 67 mg sodium.

For couscous, per serving, 340 kcals (1428 kJ), 1.5 g fat, of which saturated fat negligible, sodium, trace.

For whole meal, per serving, 623 kcals (2655 kJ), 7 g fat, of which 1 g saturated, 668 mg sodium.

Method
1 For the sauce, add a little of the juice from the tinned pineapple to the cornflour in a saucepan and mix until it makes a smooth paste. Add the rest of the juice and all the other sauce ingredients and bring to the boil. Boil for 1 minute, or until thickened.
2 If using tofu or Quorn, place the pieces in the pan with the sauce and allow to marinate. Add to the wok or pan with the sauce at step 5.
3 Gently heat the oil in a wok or large frying pan. Add the shallots, carrots, red pepper and ginger. Turn up the heat and cook for about 2 minutes, taking care that it doesn't burn. Then add the garlic and cook for a further minute.
4 If using meat, put the contents of the wok or pan into another dish temporarily, to be returned to the wok at the beginning of step 5. Cut the meat into thin strips. Stir-fry for about 3 minutes. Add a splash of water (not oil) if the wok or pan gets too dry. Prepare the couscous according to the instructions on the packet.
5 Add the remaining ingredients, apart from the sauce, and stir-fry for 2 minutes. Stir frequently or toss à la television chefs! Stir in the sauce (and tofu or Quorn, if using). Cook for 4 to 5 minutes. Add an extra splash of water if required. Serve on a bed of the couscous.

Mushroom risotto
Serves 4

This recipe was taught to one of the authors by an Italian. It uses the original method of making risotto and is cooked in such a way that the rice takes on the full flavour of the mushrooms. Serve with warm bread rolls (see pages 129–30) for a lovely light meal. *Buon appetito*!

Ingredients

2 tsp olive oil
285 g (10 oz) mushrooms,
    wiped and thickly sliced
1.2 litres (2 pints) Vegetable
    stock (page 104)
1 medium onion, finely
    chopped
1 garlic clove, crushed

340 g (12 oz) risotto rice
1 tbsp sherry
$\frac{1}{2}$ tsp grated nutmeg
few sprigs fresh parsley,
    chopped
4 tomatoes, sliced, to garnish
freshly grated Parmesan
    cheese, to serve

Nutritional analysis

Per serving, 390 kcals (1638 kJ), 6 g fat, of which 1 g saturated, 600 mg sodium.

Method

1 Heat half the oil in a large saucepan and add the mushrooms. Fry on a low heat for 3 minutes or so, then add the vegetable stock. Bring to the boil, then simmer gently for 5 minutes. Cover and remove from the heat.
2 Place the remaining oil in a large frying pan and heat. Add the chopped onion and garlic and fry over a medium heat, covered, for 5 to 6 minutes, until soft. Add the rice to the onion and garlic and fry for a couple of minutes.
3 Turn the heat down, then add 1 ladle of liquid from the stock mixture, but try not to include any of the mushrooms at this stage, just the liquid. Wait for the liquid to soak into the rice, then add another ladleful. Continue like this until all the liquid has been used and the rice is cooked.
4 Add the sherry, nutmeg, chopped parsley and mushrooms and cook the whole mixture together for a few more minutes.
5 Garnish with the tomato slices and add a sprinkling of the freshly grated Parmesan cheese on top, then serve immediately.

Home-made curry
Serves 4–6

Adjust the number of chillies to suit your own particular taste and note the advice for preparation on page 88.

Serve your curry on a bed of rice or couscous with the sorts of accompaniments we suggest for Cheat's curry (page 159), such as

Mango chutney, a cucumber and yogurt raita, lettuce and tomato side salad, together with your home-made Chapattis (page 132) and a crispy poppadom. You can buy very low-fat poppadoms with less than a gram of fat each that can be cooked in a microwave in seconds.

Ingredients

2 tsp olive oil
1 medium onion, finely chopped
2 red chillies, finely chopped
1 garlic clove, crushed or finely chopped
1 tsp ginger
2 tsp ground cumin
2 tsp ground coriander
1 tsp turmeric
1 tsp garam masala or 1–2 tbsp favourite curry powder or

paste instead of this and the above spices
1 courgette, sliced
1 medium aubergine, diced (2-cm/$\frac{3}{4}$-in cubes)
1 red pepper, diced
2 x 400-g (14-oz) tins chopped tomatoes
1 tbsp tomato ketchup
cooked lean meat or Quorn sufficient for 4 people

Nutritional analysis

For vegetable curry, per serving, 98 kcals (412 kJ), 3 g fat, of which 0.5 g saturated, 167 mg sodium.

For vegetable curry with lean meat (extra lean minced beef), per serving for 4, 228 kcals (958 kJ), 10 g fat, of which 3.5 g saturated, 235 mg sodium.

For basmati rice, per serving, 215 kcals (903 kJ), 0.3 g fat, of which saturated fat negligible, sodium, trace.

Method

1 Place the oil in a large flameproof casserole dish. Add the onion and chillies. Cover and cook over a gentle heat for 5 to 6 minutes.
2 Add the garlic and spices and cook for about 1 minute.
3 Add the courgette, aubergine and pepper and cook for a further minute.
4 Pour in the chopped tomatoes, together with the ketchup. Simmer gently, covered, for 30 minutes, or until the vegetables are tender.
5 Add the cooked meat or Quorn, if using. Bring to the boil, then turn down the heat and simmer for about 5 minutes.

Variation

Try introducing a Thai flavour by adding 1 tablespoon chopped fresh lemongrass to the other spices.

Bean goulash
Serves 4

This recipe has been very well received by readers of the companion volume, *How to Keep Your Cholesterol in Check,* and so we have reproduced it here for the benefit of people who may not have read the book. It provides a delicious meal, full of all sorts of heart-healthy ingredients. Try it with baked potatoes and a little wholegrain mustard.

Ingredients

2 tsp olive oil
1 onion, finely chopped
1 garlic clove, crushed
1 tbsp wholemeal flour
1 heaped tbsp paprika
225 g (8 oz) courgettes, sliced
2 medium carrots, sliced
1 red pepper, diced

1 x 400-g (14-oz) tin tomatoes
2 tbsp tomato purée
2 tbsp red wine
275 ml ($\frac{1}{2}$ pint) vegetable stock
1 x 400-g (14-oz) tin haricot
   or kidney beans, drained
   and rinsed

Nutritional analysis
Per serving, 178 kcals (748 kJ), 3 g fat, of which 0.5 g saturated, 596 mg sodium.
   Per dumpling (see page 96), 124 kcals (521 kJ), 3 g fat, of which 1 g saturated, 150 mg sodium.

Method
1 Preheat the oven to 180°C (350°F/gas mark 4). Then heat the oil in a flameproof casserole dish.
2 Add the onion and garlic, cover and cook gently until it has softened.
3 Stir in the flour and paprika, then add the courgettes, carrots and pepper. Stir the mixture so that the vegetables are well coated with the flour and paprika. Cook for 1 minute.
4 Add the tomatoes, purée, wine and stock. Cover and bring to the boil, stirring frequently.
5 Bake in the preheated oven for 55 minutes, or until the vegetables have softened.
6 Add the beans to the casserole and cook for a further 10 minutes.

Variation
Bean goulash with dumplings
4 heaped tbsp self-raising flour
1 level tsp dried mixed herbs
25 g (1 oz) low-fat unsaturated margarine
120 ml (4 fl oz) water

1 Mix the flour and herbs together in a mixing bowl, then rub in the margarine until the mixture resembles breadcrumbs. Add enough water to make a paste.
2 Then drop 4 tablespoon-size portions on to the top of the Bean goulash after mixing in the beans at step 6.

Ratatouille
Serves 4

It is a good idea to make double the quantity of Ratatouille and keep or freeze the extra, for Tortillas or Pancakes with Ratatouille, Cheat's curry or Vegetable or meat lasagne (pages 159–60). It is delicious, too, simply served on a bed of pasta or with a baked potato or on top of (or inside) some Naan bread.

Ingredients

1 tsp olive oil
1 medium onion, finely
  chopped
1 garlic clove, crushed
1 medium aubergine, diced
2 peppers, red or mixed
  colours, diced
2 courgettes, sliced
2 tbsp red wine
1 tbsp tomato purée
1 tbsp tomato ketchup

1 x 400-g (14-oz) tin chopped
  tomatoes
1 x 400-g (14-oz) tin red
  kidney beans in water,
  drained and rinsed (drained
  weight about 240 g/$8\frac{1}{2}$ oz)
1 tbsp fresh basil, chopped, or
  1 tsp dried
freshly ground black pepper
few sprigs fresh parsley,
  chopped, to garnish

Nutritional analysis
Per serving, 150 kcals (630 kJ), 2 g fat, of which saturated fat negligible, 373 mg sodium. Ragù meat sauce, per serving, 186 kcals (781 kJ), 5 g fat, of which 2 g saturated, 406 mg sodium.

Method
1 Add the oil to a large saucepan or flameproof casserole dish over a low heat. Stir the chopped onion into the oil and allow to soften for 5 to 6 minutes with the lid on. Add in the garlic for the last couple of minutes.
2 Stir in the rest of the ingredients, apart from the beans. Bring to the boil and allow to simmer gently with the lid on for about 20 to 30 minutes, or until the vegetables are tender. Add the beans and basil for the last 5 minutes of cooking. Season with black pepper. Serve with your chosen accompaniments, garnished with the chopped parsley.

Variation
Ragù meat sauce
This is a modified version of a traditional Italian recipe. To keep down the overall fat content, we have omitted the usual chicken livers and bacon. The sauce is suitable for use with Lasagne (pages 98–9).

To make, follow the steps above for Ratatouille, but omit the aubergine, peppers and courgettes and add 170 g (6 oz) lean minced beef at the end of step 1. Cook it for a few more minutes until the mince has browned, stirring all the time. At the end of step 2, cook the mixture gently for a further 20 minutes without the lid.

Vegetable lasagne
Serves 4

For the topping, you can buy ready-grated mozzarella cheese, and some shops also sell a reduced-fat (around 8 per cent) variety. Baked potatoes and French beans complement this lasagne perfectly.

Ingredients
For white sauce

275 ml ($\frac{1}{2}$ pint) skimmed milk	sprinkling freshly grated
1 heaped tbsp plain flour	nutmeg
1 tsp olive oil	1 bay leaf
6 black peppercorns, crushed	

For lasagne

1 x Ratatouille recipe (pages 96–7)	70 g ($2\frac{1}{2}$ oz) mozzarella cheese, grated or finely chopped
4 sheets lasagne that doesn't require precooking	

Nutritional analysis
Per serving, 317 kcals (1331 kJ), 8 g fat, of which 3 g saturated, 50 mg sodium. If use 8 per cent mozzarella, 5 g fat, of which 2 g saturated and slightly fewer calories and reduced salt.

Variation using mince, per serving, 352 kcals (1478 kJ), 10 g fat, of which 5 g saturated, or 7 g with 3 g saturated with 8 per cent mozzarella, 552 mg sodium.

Variation using roasted vegetables, per serving, 268 kcals (1126 kJ), 9 g fat, of which 3 g saturated, or 6 g with 2 g saturated with 8 per cent mozzarella, 170 mg sodium.

Method
1 Grease a 23-cm (9-in) square lasagne dish and preheat the oven to 180°C (350°F/gas mark 4).
2 Place all the ingredients for the white sauce in a saucepan and bring to the boil, stirring continuously. Simmer for a further 2 minutes, or until the sauce becomes thick and smooth, stirring throughout.
3 Prepare the Ratatouille according to the recipe and spoon half

over the base of the prepared lasagne dish, then place 2 of the sheets of lasagne, side by side on top. Pour half the white sauce over the lasagne sheets then spread the rest of the Ratatouille over the top. Place the two remaining sheets of pasta on top and cover with the rest of the white sauce and top with the grated or diced mozzarella cheese, sprinkling it evenly.

4 Bake in the preheated oven, towards the top, for 45 minutes.

Variations
Classic lasagne
For a version using lean minced beef instead of vegetables, follow the Ragù meat sauce variation of the Ratatouille recipe (pages 96–7) and substitute it for the Ratatouille in step 3.

Roasted vegetable lasagne
At step 3, instead of Ratatouille, use roasted vegetables. You will need 1 red and 1 yellow pepper, diced, 1 medium onion, 3 garlic cloves, 2 courgettes and 1 aubergine, sliced, and 12 cherry tomatoes cut in half. Season them with freshly ground black pepper, then place them in a roasting tin, drizzle with just over 1 tablespoon of olive oil and roast in the middle of a 220°C (425°F/gas mark 7) oven for 30 minutes.

Distribute 1 tablespoon of tomato purée plus 1 tablespoon of red wine over each of the two layers of lasagne sheets before pouring on the white sauce at step 3.

You can also use roasted vegetables with any sort of pasta. Topped with a little mozzarella cheese, this makes a tasty dish.

Spaghetti bolognese with Quorn mince
Serves 4

We have chosen to use Quorn mince instead of beef for this recipe as minced beef contains over five times as much fat as Quorn, with more than twice the amount of saturated fat.

If you like pasta, you could have a go at making your own. All you need are flour, eggs and water to make the dough and a pasta machine with rollers or a pasta attachment to a mixer to make various types of pasta.

This recipe was also popular when it appeared in *How to Keep*

Your Cholesterol in Check. If you are in a hurry, for a quick version of it, see the 'Meals in under 30 minutes' section. Serve either version with some Mango chutney (pages 70–1) and a side salad of lettuce, tomato and fresh basil for a tasty, filling meal.

Ingredients

2 tsp extra virgin olive oil
1 medium onion, finely chopped
1 garlic clove, crushed or finely chopped
235 g (8 oz) Quorn mince
1 tbsp fresh basil or 1 tsp dried
2 x 400-g (14-oz) tins chopped tomatoes

1 carrot, sliced
1 celery stick, chopped
2 tbsp tomato purée
2 tbsp red wine
freshly ground black pepper
225–340 g (8–12 oz) dried spaghetti
Parmesan cheese, to serve

Nutritional analysis

Per serving, 400 kcals (1680 kJ), 7 g fat, of which 2 g saturated, 320 mg sodium.

For lean mince variation, per serving, 423 kcals (1777 kJ), 7 g fat, of which 2 g saturated, 164 mg sodium.

Method

1 Heat the oil in a large frying pan or flameproof casserole dish. Add the onion, cover and cook over a low heat for 5 to 6 minutes, or until softened, stirring occasionally so it does not burn.
2 Add the garlic, Quorn mince and basil and cook for about 3 minutes.
3 Stir in the chopped tomatoes, carrot, celery, tomato purée and red wine. Season to taste with pepper. Bring to the boil and cook gently for about 30 to 35 minutes, or until the vegetables are tender.
4 Meanwhile, cook the spaghetti separately in a large pan of boiling water.
5 Drain the spaghetti, serve, then spoon the bolognese sauce on top, adding a sprinkling of Parmesan cheese.

Variations

You can use 2 tablespoons TVP (textured vegetable protein made from soya beans) instead of Quorn if you prefer.

For a meat version, use 225 g (8 oz) lean minced beef.

Vegetables and fruit

Fruit and vegetables form an essential part of a heart-healthy diet and, as we have seen, we should all aim to eat at least five portions a day (see Chapter 3). Although potatoes count as starchy foods rather than vegetables in terms of the 'five portions a day' advice, we include them here in our comments about food preparation.

Raw or cooked?

Fruit and vegetables are beneficial however we have them, providing us with a whole range of nutrients, including protein, as we have already seen in Chapters 2 and 3. You will have a better idea of exactly what you're eating with fresh produce, of course, but frozen, dried and tinned foods are all OK, as also are juices. Fruit and vegetables will generally retain more of their antioxidant properties when raw or lightly cooked, however.

Most fruits and some vegetables – carrots and celery, for example – make excellent snacks eaten raw. Fruits appear in a variety of forms, both cooked and uncooked, as ingredients in the range of delicious and easy-to-prepare desserts described later in the book. Preparing these desserts should turn eating for a healthy heart into one of life's great pleasures!

When cooking vegetables, we would recommend steaming. Different vegetables need to be steamed for different lengths of time, so you need to stagger the introduction of vegetables to the steamer according to the cooking times they need. This is easy to do in a layered steaming saucepan, but, for speed, you may prefer to cook vegetables such as potatoes in water. If you are only cooking a small amount, you can put a metal 'petal' steamer with the other vegetables in it on top of the potatoes in a pan, then cover with the lid.

Try preparing potatoes in different ways. Baked potatoes, for example, with a plain tuna filling make a good, heart-healthy lunchtime snack. New potatoes, sweet potatoes and yams are better as they have a lower glycaemic index, but any type of potato provides an important source of complex carbohydrates (see Chapter 2, pp. 6–8).

Don't feel that you must avoid roast potatoes or chips. As we have indicated earlier, it's just a matter of finding low-fat versions. For example, you can roast potatoes in a small amount of olive oil to provide a tasty and healthy accompaniment to several of our recipes.

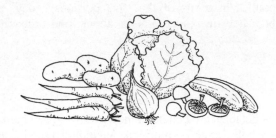

Roast potatoes
Serves 4

Ingredients
700 g (1½ lbs) medium
   potatoes, peeled
1 tbsp olive oil

Nutritional analysis
Per serving, 138 kcals (580 kJ), 1 g fat, of which saturated fat negligible, 12 mg sodium.

Method
1 Preheat the oven to 190°C (375°F/gas mark 5), then line a small baking tray with foil and drizzle the olive oil over the foil. Fill a large pan with water and bring to the boil.
2 Cut the potatoes in half and boil for 5 minutes. Drain off the water and shake the potatoes about in the pan vigorously so that the surface becomes roughened.
3 Put the prepared baking tray in the oven for 2 to 3 minutes to warm up. This allows the oil to spread over the base of the tray.

Then place the potatoes on the tray, turning them so that they become coated with oil. Bake on a high shelf for about 35 to 40 minutes, or until crisp and browned.

4 Transfer the potatoes immediately to a warmed dish so that they don't soak up the remaining oil from the baking tray. You'll be surprised to find when you remove the potatoes that at least a couple of teaspoonfuls of oil are left on the foil, so only about 1 teaspoonful has been used in the cooking.

Variation
Use an olive oil spray. Just spray the foil and the tops of the potatoes. This method also produces excellent roast potatoes.

Roast vegetables

Follow the same method as given for Roast potatoes, again using little more than a teaspoon of oil or some olive oil spray. Just put a selection of thickly sliced or chopped vegetables – onions, courgettes, peppers, aubergine, sweet potato and so on – on to a baking tray lined with a sheet of foil and bake as for potatoes. Chopped vegetables on skewers also make excellent bedfellows on the barbecue (pages 84–5).

How to chop vegetables like a professional chef
When slicing a vegetable such as a courgette, use your fingernails as a guide for the knife blade. Lie the vegetable on the chopping board and hold it where you want to cut with your middle three fingers. Then, slice down with the knife, using your nails as the guide, gradually drawing back your fingernails for each succeeding slice. You will find that the knife blade only needs to rise a fraction above the top of the vegetable for each cut and that you can produce a beautifully sliced courgette in no time at all. If you're not accustomed to using this particular chef's trick, you will need to practise a little, but you'll soon get the hang of it. We should stress that *you do need to be careful when using this technique*, but it's not really as hazardous as it sounds! Start slowly and gradually build up speed and you'll be surprised at how professional your slicing skills can become.

Vegetable stock

Makes 1 litre (1¾ pints)

Bought vegetable stock cubes or granules tend to have a very high salt content, so it's a good idea to dilute, using half the cubes or granules to the recommended water; or, better still, use this home-made stock. You can double the amounts in the recipe and freeze the extra for later use. Freeze in 275-ml (½-pint) amounts, then you can make up the 570-ml (1-pint), 850-ml (1½-pint) or 1.2-litre (2-pint) amounts required in other soup recipes (see pages 63–6). If a little short of the required stock for a recipe, just top up with water.

Ingredients

1 garlic clove, halved
225 g (8 oz) sweet potato, peeled and roughly chopped
1 medium leek
1 large onion, peeled and roughly chopped
115 g (4 oz) carrot, peeled and roughly chopped
115 g (4 oz) courgette, sliced
1 medium celery stick, roughly chopped

3 good-sized broccoli florets, halved
2 sprigs fresh flat-leaf parsley with stems, roughly chopped
1 sprig fresh thyme, stalk removed
1 bay leaf
5 black peppercorns, crushed
1.2 litres (2 pints) cold water

Nutritional analysis

Per litre (1¾ pints) clear, strained stock, negligible calories, negligible fat, negligible saturated fat, 156 mg sodium. Per 275 ml (½ pint) stock, negligible calories and fat, 43 mg sodium.

Method

1 To prepare the leek, trim a little from the top and bottom, then split in half lengthways from the top down, but don't cut through completely. Fan and rinse out the dirt between the layers under the tap before chopping.

2 Place all the ingredients in a very large saucepan or flameproof casserole dish. Cover and bring slowly to the boil. Reduce the heat to a gentle simmer. Skim off any scum, then simmer very gently with the lid on for 45 minutes, skimming from time to time, if necessary.

3 Take out the vegetables with a straining spoon and transfer to a food processor if you intend to make the Thick vegetable soup (see below). Strain out any vegetables left using a sieve and transfer them to the food processor, too, leaving the clear vegetable stock. Allow to cool. Pour 425 ml ($\frac{3}{4}$ pint) of the stock into a jug for the soup recipe below and freeze the remaining liquid (roughly 570 ml/1 pint), in a plastic container for later use.

Thick vegetable soup
Serves 4

If you are making double quantities of the Vegetable stock and you intend to make this soup, simply double the quantities for the soup recipe, too. It freezes well, so, if you don't need 8 servings, freeze the rest for a later occasion.

Ingredients

425ml ($\frac{3}{4}$ pint) Vegetable stock (page 104)
vegetables from making Vegetable stock
1 tbsp tomato purée

juice of $\frac{1}{2}$ lemon
1 tbsp white wine
2 pinches chilli powder
freshly ground black pepper

Nutritional analysis
Per serving, 110 kcals (462 kJ), 1 g fat, of which saturated fat negligible, 51 mg sodium.

Method
1 Make the stock as directed in the recipe, straining out the vegetables and putting them into a blender. Remove the bay leaf and process the vegetables very briefly (no more than 5 seconds), leaving a nice bit of texture in the mixture.
2 Pour into a large saucepan or flameproof casserole and add the vegetable stock, together with the tomato purée, lemon juice, white wine and chilli powder. Boil for 10 minutes, then simmer for a further 20 minutes. Season to taste with black pepper and serve with warm rolls.

The heart-health benefits of different sorts of vegetables

We have discussed the benefits of various vegetables in Chapters 2 and 3, but here are a few reminders plus some additions.

- Vegetables, like fruit, act as an antioxidant police force, being particularly good sources of the ACE vitamins.
- Vitamin A is converted by our bodies from beta-carotene, the pigment that gives many plant foods their green, yellow and orange colours. It's found in especially good quantities in dark green leafy vegetables, such as spinach, watercress and broccoli, and in carrots and red peppers.
- Vegetables, like fruit, are a good source of vitamin C – especially broccoli, greens, parsley, peppers and new potatoes.
- Leafy green vegetables also provide a good supply of vitamin E, together with vegetable oils. Nuts, too, provide us with such oils.
- Tomatoes are an excellent source of all the ACE vitamins and contain another potent antioxidant called lycopene.
- Omega-3 fatty acids, which help, for example, to prevent the blood from getting too sticky (pages 10–12) are found in sweet potatoes, spinach, leafy green vegetables and pumpkins.
- Pulses, as we have seen, are excellent sources of soluble fibre. They have some of the lowest scores on the glycaemic index of all foods and, because of their value in heart-healthy cooking, we have included a special section on the range of pulses available and how to prepare them.

Using pulses

Pulses (beans, peas and lentils) are among the most versatile varieties of vegetable used in cooking. They are *nutrient dense*, which means that they provide plenty of nutrients, such as protein, iron, zinc, calcium, folate and soluble fibre. They are also a rich source of some important health-promoting substances called phytoestrogens, some of which have anti-inflammatory, antiviral, antifungal and antibacterial properties and others have been shown to protect against the development of cancer and raised blood pressure. Similarly, beans generally are high in folate, which lowers the level of homocysteine in the blood and reduces the risk of cardiovascular disease. Soya beans in particular are a good source of the essential omega-3 fatty acids, so lots of our recipes include soya beans, soya milk and soya bean curd (tofu).

Pulses are also:

- cheap
- free of saturated fat
- low in calories
- have a low glycaemic index rating
- filling.

You will find plenty of recipes using pulses in this book. Try the Bean goulash, for example (pages 95–6), or the lentil-based soups (page 155).

Basic preparation methods for dried pulses

Essentially, dried pulses need to be *soaked* first and then *cooked*, but you will need to pay particular attention to the instructions as different varieties will require slight variations in method.

Soaking

Place the dried pulses in a saucepan and cover with two to three times their volume of cold water. Soak overnight or during the day. As a shortcut, you can rinse the pulses, add three times their volume of water, bring to the boil, boil for two to three minutes, then remove from the heat and allow to soak for an hour. Drain, add fresh water and cook as usual.

Cooking

Drain off the soaking water. Never cook the pulses in the water they have been soaked in – the substances that leach from the pulses into the water used during preparation contribute to flatulence! Add two to three times their volume of fresh water. Don't add salt to the cooking water. Apart from being potentially hazardous to heart health, it slows down water absorption so the cooking takes longer and the pulses are tougher. Bring to the boil then simmer until tender. Follow the directions on the packet or the information below for specific varieties of pulse as a guide to how much time they take to cook.

Some useful tips

- If you haven't time to soak and cook dried pulses, use tinned and vacuum-packed versions. One 400-g (14-oz) tin of beans substitutes for $\frac{3}{4}$ cup of dried beans (100 g/$3\frac{1}{2}$ oz).
- Precook your own dried pulses and freeze them in small batches.
- Soaked or cooked beans can be kept for several days in the fridge.

Different pulses and how to cook them

Chickpeas (also known as garbanzo beans) These large, caramel-coloured legumes are popular in Middle Eastern and Mediterranean dishes. You can buy them either dried or in tins.

Cover dried chickpeas with plenty of cold water and soak overnight. Drain, then put them in a saucepan and cover with clean water. Bring to the boil, cook for 10 minutes, then simmer gently for $1\frac{1}{2}$ hours, until tender.

Red kidney beans These are the red beans you find in Mexican dishes, such as chilli con carne and tacos. They can also be added to mince dishes and they form the basis of the Bean goulash recipe (pages 95–6).

The dried beans need to be soaked overnight, then drained, rinsed and fresh water added. Bring to the boil and boil vigorously for about 15 minutes, then simmer for 1 to $1\frac{1}{2}$ hours. It's important to cook these beans thoroughly, so don't be tempted to shorten the cooking time!

Split peas Green or yellow split peas are great to add to soups and will cook in about 40 minutes without presoaking. Green split peas are traditionally used in pea and ham soup.

Lentils Lentils are available in whole green or brown, whole red or split red varieties. The split lentils are relatively quick to cook, needing to simmer, partly covered, for only 10 to 15 minutes, without presoaking. The dried whole lentils, though, need to be boiled for about 45 minutes.

Cannellini beans These are small white beans, available dried or in tins.

The dried beans need to be soaked overnight, drained and rinsed. Add fresh water, boil for 15 minutes, then allow to simmer for 1 to $1\frac{1}{2}$ hours, until tender.

Onions and garlic

We have the Romans to thank for these excellent, heart-healthy cooking ingredients, When they invaded Britain, they introduced onions into our diet.

The traditional type of onion is called *Allium cepa*. The red or whitish varieties are probably better for using in raw dishes than the brown onion, as they tend to be sweeter in their natural state. Try large, mild Spanish onions, spring onions or shallots (*Allium ascalonicum*).

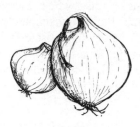

As we saw in Chapter 3, onions are good sources of flavonoids – the potent antioxidant substances – and they are especially rich in one called quercetin. They help to protect us from problems such as raised cholesterol and triglyceride levels, which increase our susceptibility to heart disease. Studies have also shown that consumption of onions tends to be associated with lower blood pressure, less sticky blood and lower blood sugar levels, as well as a reduced incidence of certain forms of asthma and cancer.

How to chop onions

Many of our recipes contain instructions for good-sized onions to be 'finely chopped'. You may prefer to use a food processor, but, if not, try the following – with care!

1 Slice the onion in half lengthways.
2 Lay the cut surface of one half face down on the chopping board and cut the onion into several thin slices. Try to hold together the shape of the onion half while slicing.
3 Make a couple of horizontal cuts across the onion, taking care not to produce additional finger slices!

4 Turn the onion through 90 degrees and then cut into fine slices as before, but this time across the previous cuts. You will find that the onion will now disintegrate into the finely chopped pieces you require.

Garlic

Garlic is another member of the onion family. It has a long history of use in cooking and herbal medicine and many of the traditional claims that have been made for its health-giving properties have been substantiated by medical research. Garlic contains antioxidants and studies have shown that it can help to reduce fibrinogen, triglyceride and LDL levels, while increasing the good HDL cholesterol. It also has the anticoagulant properties of its onion relatives and appears to help fight bacteria.

If you are crushing garlic using a garlic press, try crushing the clove without peeling it – it's much easier to clean the garlic press afterwards as the peel just lifts out in one go.

Fruit

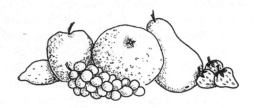

Any type of fruit is a heart-healthy option. Here are some good reasons for using plenty of fruit in your cooking.

- Fruits such as apples and pears, grapes, citrus fruits – oranges, satsumas, clementines, lemons, limes, grapefruit, ugli fruit – and dried fruits – figs, dates, apricots and raisins – help to provide fibre, particularly soluble fibre, which can contribute to lowering cholesterol levels in the blood.
- Orange or deep yellow fruits, such as apricots, mangoes and cantaloupe melons, help the body maintain its levels of vitamin A.

- Fruits are the star providers of vitamin C and top among these are blackcurrants, strawberries, raspberries, kiwi fruit, mangoes and papayas.
- Plums contain vitamin E, another of the ACE group of vitamins.
- Bananas and dried fruit help to regulate blood pressure by providing us with potassium, as do plums and, in their dried state, prunes.

So, think fruit when planning meals. Why not try some of the more exotic fruits available everywhere today?

Carambola or star fruit

This is a greeny yellow fruit and both the skin and flesh are edible. Its attractive star shape makes it an excellent garnish for cold meats or for use in salads. You can use it in a stir-fry or simply enjoy it sliced as a snack. The slices freeze well, too.

Carambola are rich in vitamin A and potassium, as well as containing good amounts of vitamin C and calcium.

Guava

Scoop out the seeds and serve the flesh with yogurt. It can also be added to fruit salads.

Guavas are rich in vitamins A and C, potassium and calcium.

Kiwi fruit

Unripe kiwi fruit can be stored in a fridge for up to a month or more as they keep very well. Kiwi fruit are rich in vitamin C, iron and calcium.

Peel and cut them into slices for a nice, decorative garnish or scoop out the edible flesh and small seeds. Eat this raw with yogurt or breakfast cereals or use slices in fruit salads or as a garnish for fish patés, cold meats or with low-fat (5 per cent or less) cream cheese.

Mango

Mangoes contain vitamins A, B and C and are high in potassium.

This succulent fruit forms the basis of the delicious Mango chutney recipe (pages 70–1), but is delicious eaten raw. Use in fruit salads, fools (pages 123–5) or cool, refreshing drinks or water ices (page 147).

To test for ripeness, press the outer skin – it should give a little. If you are using the mango for a fruit salad, an easy way to cut it into neat cubes is to first, without peeling, slice off each side just grazing the stone. Then, take each slice and cut the flesh into a lattice of small squares without cutting through the skin. Finally, take hold of the slice at each end and turn it inside out so that the cubes stick out and are easily cut off.

Papaya (paw-paw)

The papaya contains vitamins A and C, potassium and calcium.

Try scooping out the seeds, sprinkling a little lime juice on top and eating it on its own. You can also use it in a vegetable or pork stir-fry (pages 91–2) or try the attractive dessert recipe below.

Papaya with grapes and cream
Serves 2

This makes a delicious dessert and is ready in minutes. Also, a papaya will not lose its colour after cutting, so you can prepare it in advance without worrying that it will spoil.

Ingredients
1 papaya and 1 lime
2 tbsp Quark and yogurt cream
  (page 113)

handful seedless grapes

Nutritional analysis
Per serving, 144 kcals (60.5 kJ), negligible fat, 29 mg sodium.

Method
1 Cut the papaya in half lengthways, scoop out the seeds and discard.
2 Squeeze a little lime juice over the flesh and then fill the space left by the seeds with the Quark and yogurt cream. Place the seedless grapes on top.

Passion fruit

Like the papaya, passion fruit contains plenty of vitamin A, along with vitamin C, potassium and calcium.

When the skin becomes wrinkled, the fruit is ripe. Cut it in half and scoop out the flesh and seeds. Purée and use it in sorbets, fools or smoothies (page 123–5) or add the juice to drinks.

Experiment with fruit

Fruit of all kinds provides the basis for many of the recipes in this book. On page 115, for example, there is a recipe for Fresh fruit salad that uses mango, melon, apple, orange, kiwi fruit and grapes. We suggest, however, that you try your own versions using some of the fruit we have just described or other fruits that you have discovered. Experiment and enjoy the experience. You can congratulate yourself on having made a good, heart-healthy dessert.

To accompany your fruit dish, you could try this deliciously creamy topping. It uses quark, which is a bit like cottage cheese but smoother in texture. The variety made with skimmed milk is virtually fat free and, when mixed with a low-fat yogurt, it takes on a lovely creamy flavour.

Quark and yogurt cream
Serves 2

The ingredients given here make sufficient cream to accompany a dessert for two people. Simply add extra in the same proportions for more people.

Compared with full-fat double cream, which might have around 50 per cent fat, this cream has under 1 per cent fat per serving.

Ingredients

2 heaped tbsp quark	1 tsp honey
2 level tbsp low-fat natural bio yogurt (less than 5 per cent fat)	

Nutritional analysis

Per serving, 75 kcals (315 kJ), negligible fat, negligible saturated fat, 58 mg sodium.

Method

1 Place the quark in a bowl together with the low-fat yogurt.
2 Add the honey and mix together.

Meringues
Makes 8

Meringues usually have a very high sugar content, but here's a low-sugar version made with egg white left over from making the mince-pie pastry (pages 144–5). They are delicious served with yogurt as an accompaniment to Fresh fruit salad (page 115).

Ingredients
1 large egg white
25 g (1 oz) caster sugar

Nutritional analysis
Per meringue, 120 kcals (504 kJ), negligible fat, 67 mg sodium.

Method
1 Line a baking tray with baking parchment and preheat the oven to 100°C (200°F/gas mark $\frac{1}{4}$. Place the egg white in a mixing bowl and whisk for a minute or so with an electric hand-held whisk until the mixture stands up in stiff peaks.
2 Sift in the caster sugar. (At 3 g of added sugar per meringue, this is about half to a quarter of the usual sugar content for meringues, but it's quite sufficient.) Whisk for a few seconds until it stiffens again – the peaks don't need to be as stiff as before. Then, place 8 blobs of the mixture (about a dessertspoonful each) on to the prepared baking tray. Bake in the preheated oven for 2 hours, then turn the oven off, leave the door ajar and allow the meringues to crisp up in the oven for a further 30 minutes. Store in an airtight tin or plastic container.

Desserts

Some of the best and healthiest desserts are also often the simplest to prepare.

Fresh fruit salad
Serves 4–6

This refreshing salad is full of heart-healthy antioxidants.

You can serve it on its own or with crème fraîche, yogurt, low-fat ice-cream or Quark and yogurt cream (page 113). Alternatively, enjoy it with a Meringue (page 114) made from the egg whites left over from making pastry.

Ingredients
1 ripe galia melon, about
  1 kg/2¼ lbs
1 good-sized mango, about
  350 g/12 oz, peeled and
  diced (see method described
  on page 112)
1 large orange or 2
  clementines, peeled and
  chopped, any pips removed
115 g (4 oz) black seedless
  grapes, halved

1 kiwi fruit, peeled and sliced
extra orange juice (fresh or
  carton), if necessary
1 red apple, chopped and
  added just before serving, to
  prevent browning
sprig of fresh mint, to garnish
pinch ground ginger for each
  serving

Nutritional analysis
Per serving, 128 kcals (538 kJ), negligible fat, 48 mg sodium.

Method
1 Scoop out the flesh from the melon with a melon baller or spoon or else cut it into small chunks and place in a large serving bowl with the diced mango, orange pieces and grapes. Squeeze extra juice out of the melon shell into the bowl and place the kiwi slices on top of the fruit salad. Add extra orange juice if the salad seems too dry.
2 Chill until ready to serve and then mix in the chopped apple. Top each portion with a sprig of the mint and a pinch of ground ginger.

Chocolate and pear puddings with chocolate sauce
Makes 6

Chocolate is often seen as being off the menu in terms of a heart-healthy diet. It's true that chocolate tends to be high in fat, but it generally derives from cocoa butter, which consists of stearic acid and this is converted by our bodies into good monounsaturated fat. Chocolate also contains lots of vitamins and minerals, bioactive compounds that may be mood-lifting and substances called flavonoids, which have protective antioxidant properties. So, in moderation, chocolate's not all bad!

Serve with the chocolate sauce (the recipe here serves two, so triple it if you are serving all six puddings) and a spoonful of yogurt as desserts, or as muffins. The puddings also freeze very well, so if six are not required immediately, freeze the surplus to use later.

Ingredients
For puddings

85 g (3 oz) self-raising flour	3 tbsp semi-skimmed milk
1 heaped tbsp drinking chocolate	25 g (1 oz) caster sugar
1 heaped tsp baking powder	1 large ripe pear or 2 medium, peeled and diced (about 115 g/4 oz prepared)
1 egg	
4 tsp rapeseed oil	

For chocolate sauce

2 heaped tsp custard powder	1 level tsp sugar
2 heaped tsp drinking chocolate	200 ml ($\frac{1}{3}$ pint) semi-skimmed or soya milk

Nutritional analysis
Per pudding, without sauce, 132 kcals (554 kJ), 4 g fat, of which 1 g saturated, 160 mg sodium.

Per pudding with sauce, 245 kcals (1029 kJ), 6 g fat, of which 2 g saturated, 260 mg sodium.

Method
1 First, make the pudding. Preheat the oven to 170°C (325°F/gas mark 3), then sift the flour, drinking chocolate and baking powder together into a mixing bowl.
2 Mix together the egg, oil, milk and sugar in another bowl. Don't beat, just mix. This recipe needs gentle handling!

3 Sift the dry ingredients again into the liquid ingredients and fold together gently with a large spoon. Again, don't beat or stir, just blend swiftly – for about 30 seconds or so. Fold in the pear pieces.
4 Spoon the mixture immediately into 6 paper muffin cases or use a muffin baking tray, putting about 1 tablespoon of mixture in each case.
5 Bake on a high shelf in the preheated oven for 15 minutes.
6 While the puddings are baking, prepare the chocolate sauce. Place the custard powder, drinking chocolate and sugar into a pan. Add the milk slowly and mix to a smooth paste. Bring to the boil slowly, stirring all the time. Cook for a further 2 minutes.
7 Alternatively, you can make the sauce in the microwave. Mix the ingredients into a smooth paste in a glass jug. Place in the microwave, set on high for about $2\frac{1}{2}$ minutes or until the liquid rises to the top of the jug. Stir and return to the microwave for a further 1 minute or until the sauce rises to the top. Stir, leave for 1 minute, then pour over the puddings, set on warmed plates.

Brandy sauce
Serves 4

Delicious with Christmas pudding (pages 118–19), this sauce is very low in fat and easy to make.

Ingredients
2 tbsp cornflour   brandy, to taste
1 tbsp sugar
600 ml (approximately 1 pint)
   skimmed milk

Nutritional analysis
Per serving, 150 kcals (630 kJ), negligible fat, 90 mg sodium.

Method
1 Mix the cornflour and sugar in a non-stick saucepan. Add the milk a little at a time until it forms a smooth paste.
2 Bring the mixture slowly to the boil on a low heat, stirring continuously. Cook gently for 2–3 minutes.
3 Remove from the heat and stir in brandy to taste.

Christmas pudding
Makes 1-kg ($2\frac{1}{4}$-lb) pudding, yielding 12–14 slices

Traditional Christmas puddings are often made with beef suet – the layer of fat found around the animal's kidneys and loins, which consists of 87 per cent total fat, of which 48 per cent is saturated. Our version uses a little low-fat, low-salt margarine instead of suet and includes lots of antioxidant goodies. Allow to mature for a few weeks before reheating and serving.

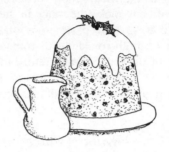

Ingredients

140 g (5 oz) dried mixed fruit, with peel

140 g (5 oz) sultanas

25 g (1 oz) ready-to-eat dates, roughly chopped

50 g (2 oz) glacé cherries, quartered

50 g (2 oz) soft light brown sugar

3 tsp mixed spice

1 tsp ground ginger

zest of $\frac{1}{2}$ an orange + 2 tbsp orange juice

2 tbsp sherry or brandy

50 g (2 oz) wholemeal self-raising flour

115 g (4 oz) breadcrumbs

50 g (2 oz) walnuts, roughly chopped

25 g (1 oz) flaked almonds

115 g (4 oz) carrots, grated

1 medium cooking apple (approximately 225 g/8 oz) peeled, cored and grated

40 g ($1\frac{1}{2}$ oz) low-fat unsaturated margarine

1 egg, mixed with 1 tbsp skimmed milk

Nutritional analysis
Per slice, 192 kcals (806 kJ), 6 g fat, of which 1 g saturated, 88 mg sodium.

Method

1 Mix together the dried mixed fruit, sultanas, dates, cherries, sugar and spices. Add the orange zest and juice, sherry or brandy, stir well, then leave to soak, covered, overnight.

2 Grease a 1-litre (2-pint) pudding basin or two 500-ml (1-pint) basins really well. Mix the flour, breadcrumbs and nuts in a large bowl. Then stir in the soaked fruit mixture, together with the grated apple and carrots. Finally, add the margarine and egg and milk mixture. Mix well.

3 Place the mixture in the prepared pudding basin or basins. It should fill it or come to within about 2.5 cm (1 in) of the top. Then, cover with greaseproof paper and a piece of foil, making a pleat in each to allow for expansion. Secure the foil with a strong elastic band and then tie down with string.

4 When ready to cook, either steam or use a pressure cooker. Steam for 4 hours in 2 litres ($3\frac{1}{2}$ pints) of water, topping up with boiling water as necessary. Steam for another 3 hours before serving.
OR
Place in a pressure cooker, bring to the boil, cover and steam (on simmer) without pressure for 30 minutes in $1\frac{3}{4}$ litres (approximately 3 pints) of water. Then, cook at high pressure for $2\frac{1}{2}$ hours. Reheat for 30 minutes at high pressure in 875 ml (approximately $1\frac{1}{2}$ pints) of boiling water before serving with custard, Quark and yogurt cream (page 113) or Brandy sauce (page 117).

Blackberry and apple crumble
Serves 6

This recipe uses a topping in which the quantity of fat and sugar is considerably reduced compared with traditional crumble recipes – it is both heart-healthy and tasty.

You can use this crumble recipe (or your own version of it) with any number of fruits – apples, pears, plums, cherries – or combinations of fruits, as we have done here. Use fruits as they come into season or try the dried variety out of season. We suggest using about 700 g (just over $1\frac{1}{2}$ lbs) of prepared fruit. The amount should be enough to fill most of the dish, but leave space for the crumble topping. If you overfill it, you'll find that the mixture will spill out of the dish during baking. You may need to adjust the water content for some recipes, and with less sweet fruits you may need a little more sugar (adding eating apples to recipes helps to reduce the amount required).

Ingredients
For crumble topping

40 g (1½ oz) low-fat unsaturated margarine

40 g (1½ oz) demerara sugar

85 g (3 oz) wholemeal self-raising flour

25 g (1 oz) oats (ordinary or jumbo)

25 g (1 oz) flaked almonds

Fruit

900 g (2 lbs) eating apples, peeled, cored, finely sliced (625 g/1 lb 6 oz) prepared weight

75 g (2½ oz) blackberries, washed and drained

1 tsp demerara sugar

150 ml (¼ pint) boiling water

Nutritional analysis
Per serving, 180 kcals (756 kJ), 6 g fat, of which 1 g saturated, 47 mg sodium.

Method

1 Preheat the oven to 180°C (350°F/gas mark 4) and grease a 23-cm (9-in) diameter, 4-cm (1½-in) deep ovenproof dish. Melt the margarine and sugar in a saucepan over a low heat.

2 Stir in the flour, oats and almonds. The mixture will be dry and crunchy.

3 Cover the base of the prepared dish with apple slices. Distribute the blackberries over the top of the apples. Add the boiling water – using boiling water helps to make sure that the apples will be well cooked during baking. Then sprinkle the sugar over the fruit.

4 Cover the fruit with the crumble topping. Leave the mixture loose and crumbly on top – don't be tempted to firm it down.

5 Bake on the middle shelf of the preheated oven for 40–45 minutes. Serve with custard or Quark and yogurt cream (page 113).

Variation
Rhubarb, apple and ginger crumble
Use 700 g (just over $1\frac{1}{2}$ lbs) prepared fruit, half rhubarb and half eating apples. You will need something like 450 g (1 lb) apples weighed before peeling and coring to get 350 g apple flesh. Slice the apples and cut the rhubarb into chunks. Add 1 level tsp ground ginger to the crumble mixture at step 2 and 1 extra tsp sugar at step 3.

Pear sorbet
Serves 4

If you've got a mixer and a freezer or a freezer compartment in your fridge, you can make sorbets with fruit of all kinds, including fresh, frozen or tinned fruit. When using 'pippy' fruit, such as raspberries or blackberries, though, sieve the fruit after mixing in step 1. You may also need to add a little more sugar or honey with some fruits.

Ingredients
1 × 400-g (14-oz) tin pears in juice
1 tsp lemon juice
1 tsp sugar

handful seedless white grapes, to garnish
4 sprigs fresh mint, to garnish

Nutritional analysis
Per serving Pear sorbet, 38 kcal (160 kJ), negligible fat, 3 mg sodium. Per serving Strawberry sorbet (page 122), 62 kcals (260 kJ), negligible fat, 7 mg sodium.

Method
1 Place the whole contents of the tin into a food processor, together with the lemon juice and sugar. Mix until smooth.
2 Freeze in a suitable plastic container with a lid until it has become almost frozen and has a sorbet-like consistency. This may take 3–4 hours. Then, return it to the food processor and mix for about 2–3 seconds only. If you mix it any longer it will become too soft.
3 Transfer with a spoon or ice-cream scoop to serving dishes. Add a few seedless white grapes and decorate with a sprig of mint. Also goes nicely with a sponge finger or wafer.

Variation
Strawberry sorbet
Mix 25 g (1 oz) caster sugar with 5 tablespoons water, 1 teaspoon lemon juice and 1 teaspoon honey in a saucepan. Bring to the boil slowly. Simmer gently for 5 to 6 minutes, stirring frequently, until the mixture reduces to about 2 tablespoons of syrupy liquid. Remove from the heat. Purée 400 g (14 oz) fresh or frozen strawberries in a food processor. Add the syrupy liquid from the saucepan and mix until smooth. Then follow steps 2 and 3 as for Pear sorbet. If using frozen fruit, you will only need to refreeze for about half an hour at step 2.

Cherry yogurt slice with cream
Makes 10–12 slices

The cherry slice can be eaten as a dessert or as a cake. It is very simple to make and surprisingly rewarding for such a small amount of effort.

Note that the cream and topping ingredients serve two people, so simply multiply to cater for the number of people sharing this lovely dessert.

Ingredients
For cherry yogurt slice
225 g (8 oz) self-raising flour
1 level tsp baking powder
25 g (1 oz) sugar
2 tsp honey
1 125-g (4½-oz) carton low-fat
 black cherry yogurt
2 tbsp light olive oil

40 g (1½ oz) low-fat
 unsaturated margarine
1 egg
50 g (2 oz) glacé cherries, cut
 into eighths
3 tbsp skimmed milk
1 tsp vanilla essence

For cream and topping

2 heaped tbsp quark

2 level tbsp low-fat (less than
   5 per cent) natural yogurt

1 tsp honey

2 tbsp fresh cherries in season
   or 1×400-g (14-oz) tin
   stoned black cherries (tin
   yields 8 tbsp)

Nutritional analysis

Per slice, 146 kcals (613 kJ), 4 g fat, of which 1 g saturated, 160 mg sodium.

Per serving cream and topping, 80 kcals (336 kJ), negligible fat, 52 g sodium.

Method

1 To make the cherry yogurt slice, first grease a 900-g (2-lb) loaf tin well and preheat the oven to 170°C (325°F/gas mark 3).

2 Sift the flour and baking powder into a large bowl. Add the sugar and mix, then add the rest of the ingredients. Mix together well. The mixture will have a sticky, glutinous feel to it, but don't worry – that's how it should be.

3 Transfer the contents to the prepared loaf tin and bake on the middle shelf of the preheated oven for about 35 minutes. Then turn out on to a wire rack and allow to cool.

4 To make the cream, mix the quark with the yogurt and honey.

5 Serve the cherry yogurt slice cold topped with 2 tablespoons of the cream and 1 tbsp of the cherries.

Mango and banana fool
Serves 6

The fools will keep in the fridge for a couple of days. The mixture also freezes well – unfreeze it just long enough to reach your preferred consistency before serving to make a lovely ice-cold dessert.

If you like fools, try making your own versions with your own favourite fruits. Have fun experimenting!

Ingredients

3 ripe mangoes (about
  1 kg/2¼ lbs in total, 600g/
  1lb 5 oz prepared weight)
2 bananas (about 300 g/10½ oz)
  chopped
juice of 1 lime
1 heaped tbsp custard powder
275 ml (½ pint) semi-skimmed
  or soya milk

2 tsp sugar
2 tbsp low-fat yogurt
1 tbsp flaked almonds, to
  garnish
handful white seedless grapes,
  halved, to garnish

Nutritional analysis
Mango and banana fool, per serving, 164 kcals (689 kJ), 2 g fat, of which saturated fat negligible, 49 mg sodium.

Method
1 Peel the mangoes with a potato peeler, then slice off the flesh around the stone and cut into chunks. Place the mango chunks and bananas slices and lime juice in a food processor or blender. Mix to form a purée then spoon into a mixing bowl.
2 Mix the custard powder into a smooth paste with a little of the milk and half the sugar in a jug. Then stir in the remainder of the milk and heat on high in a microwave for 2½ minutes, or until the custard comes to the top of the jug. Stir and cook for a further 1 minute or until it reaches the top of the jug. Alternatively, make the custard in a saucepan by heating gently and stirring until it has thickened.
3 Allow to cool slightly, then stir the custard into the mango purée and mix together. Chill in the fridge for 2 hours. Finally, mix in the yogurt, then spoon into 6 small bowls or glasses. Sprinkle the flaked almonds over the top, together with a few of the grapes.

Variation
Apple and rhubarb fool
Peel, core and slice 1 kg (2¼ lbs) eating apples (600 g/1 lb 5 oz prepared weight) and chop 300 g (10½ oz) rhubarb and place in a saucepan. Add 25 g (1 oz) sugar, ½ teaspoon ground ginger and 1 tablespoon water, cover and cook gently until soft (about 15 minutes). Stir frequently to prevent burning. Whizz in a food processor to form a purée. Follow steps 2 and 3 to finish.

Nutritional analysis
Apple and rhubarb fool, per serving, 122 kcals (512 kJ), 2 g fat, of which saturated fat negligible, 51 mg sodium.

Apricot cheesecake
Serves 6

Cheesecakes are often very high in fat, but this recipe (a *How to Keep Your Cholesterol in Check* original) offers a tasty low-fat version. Made with yogurt and virtually fat-free quark, it provides a delicious, heart-healthy cheesecake experience. Not only that, but honey is a good source of antioxidants so, by using it in baking, we not only provide an effective sweetening ingredient but also help to keep harmful free radicals at bay.

The baked cheesecake base freezes very well, so why not make two or three at a time and freeze them? Simply defrost when required and you can whip up a delicious cheesecake in a flash.

Ingredients

50 g (2 oz) self-raising flour
25 g (1 oz) oats
25 g (1 oz) demerara sugar
1 tsp cinnamon
15 g ($\frac{1}{2}$ oz) flaked almonds
25 g (1 oz) unsaturated
 margarine
1 tbsp red wine or orange
 juice if preferred, plus 1
 extra tsp, if necessary

1 × 250-g (9-oz) tub quark
5 tbsps low-fat, bio yogurt
2 tsp honey
zest of $\frac{1}{2}$ orange, plus 1 tsp
 juice
115 g (4 oz) ready-to-eat
 apricots, chopped
small bunch of white seedless
 grapes, to serve

Nutritional analysis
Per serving (both recipes), 200 kcals (840 kJ), 6 g fat, of which 1 g saturated, 109 mg sodium.

Method
1 Grease an 18-cm (7-in) loose-based flan tin and preheat the oven to 190°C (375°F/gas mark 5).
2 Blend together the flour, oats, sugar, cinnamon and almonds (reserving a few to decorate the top of the cheesecake later) in a food processor or mixer.

3 Add the margarine and wine or orange juice and mix together. Form the pastry into a ball with your hands. Add a little more flour if it is too moist, or use an extra teaspoon of wine or orange juice if it is too dry. Place on a well floured surface and roll out to form a circle that will cover the bottom of the flan tin. Transfer it to the tin using a fish slice and mould the pastry into the base with your fingers.

4 Prick the base with a fork and bake blind in the preheated oven for 20 minutes. Then, allow it to cool and meanwhile prepare the filling.

5 In a bowl, mix together the quark, yogurt, honey, orange zest and juice and chopped apricots, reserving a small handful of pieces to decorate the top of the cheesecake later.

6 Spoon the mixture out of the bowl and on to the pastry base. Decorate the top with the reserved almonds and apricot pieces. Turn out on to a serving plate. Serve with a few white seedless grapes on each plate.

Variation
Summer fruit cheesecake
Try fresh or frozen summer fruits instead of apricots. You can buy the frozen variety at any time of the year. Select 115 g (4 oz) small fruits (black or redcurrants, raspberries, blackberries) and defrost. Pour off the liquid (save to drizzle around the slices when serving), sprinkle 1 teaspoon of sugar over the fruit and substitute it for the apricots in step 5.

Apple and cranberry cake
Serves 12

This recipe is full of antioxidants. Cranberries are rich in antioxidants and also have antibacterial properties which may help to prevent gum disease, ulcers and urinary tract infections.

Cranberries are combined with the heart-healthy apple to make a delightfully fruity, health-promoting dessert that can be served hot or cold or eaten as a tea-time cake.

Ingredients

225 g (8 oz) self-raising flour
1 tsp baking powder
1 tsp mixed spice
100 g ($3\frac{1}{2}$ oz) low-fat
    unsaturated margarine
85 g (3 oz) demerara sugar
2 eggs, beaten

2 tbsp skimmed milk
50 g (2 oz) dried cranberries,
    washed
2 medium eating apples (about
    250 g/9 oz), peeled, cored
    and sliced
1 tsp honey

Nutritional analysis
Per slice, 148 kcals (622 kJ), 5 g fat, of which 1 g saturated, 177 mg sodium.

Method

1 Grease a 20-cm (8-in) cake tin and line with greaseproof paper. Preheat the oven to 190°C (375°F/gas mark 5).
2 Sift the flour, baking powder and mixed spice into a large mixing bowl. Add the margarine and rub together or mix until the mixture resembles fine breadcrumbs.
3 To the beaten eggs add the milk, then stir into the flour mixture with two-thirds of the sugar, mixing well.
4 Spread out half the stiff cake mix in the bottom of the tin, then add half the cranberries and enough apple slices to cover the mixture, reserving the rest of the fruit for topping. Sprinkle the remaining sugar on top of the fruit.
5 Spoon the rest of the mixture over the sugared fruit. Smooth the top, then add the reserved apples and cranberries, lightly pressing them into the mixture.
6 Bake in the middle of the preheated oven for about 45 minutes, or until a skewer inserted into the cake comes out clean.
7 Allow to cool then remove from the tin and brush the top with the honey. Serve with Quark and yogurt cream (page 113).

Variation
Blueberry and apple cake
Replace the cranberries with blueberries – classified as one of the top antioxidant fruits by nutritional experts – for a tasty change.

Breads, cakes and biscuits

You will be able to find shop-bought cakes and biscuits that have acceptable levels of fat and sugar, but, if you bake your own, you are in control. You don't have to check for hidden fats because you know exactly how much you have used.

As far as bread is concerned, the main problem with the shop-bought varieties tends to be the high quantity of salt they may contain.

If you fancy trying your hand at breadmaking, it's relatively straightforward nowadays with the availability of sachets of fast-acting dried yeast. The granules, which also usually contain vitamin C, are added directly to the flour without needing to be reconstituted. All you need is some hand-hot water, a bit of stylish kneading and then some patience as you wait for the dough to rise. If you're put off by the amount of kneading, you can shorten this by using a mixer with a dough hook or leave it to one of the remarkably effective breadmaking machines you can buy. With one that has a timer, you can put the ingredients into the breadmaker before you go to bed and wake up to the smell of freshly baked bread for breakfast!

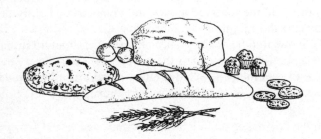

Basic bread recipe

Makes two 450-g/1-lb loaves or 12–15 good-sized rolls

Apart from the usual loaves and rolls, you can experiment with making smaller oval or baguette-shaped loaves, with diagonal cuts for decoration – just bake them in the same way as the rolls.

Ingredients

300 g (10½ oz) strong white flour

300 g (10½ oz) strong wholemeal flour

1 × 7-g sachet fast-acting dried yeast

1 tbsp rapeseed or light olive oil

about 425 ml (¾ pint) hand-hot water – a good tip is to mix 150 ml (¼ pint) boiling with 275 ml (½ pint) cold water

extra flour for dusting

a little skimmed milk, for brushing loaves/rolls

Nutritional analysis

Per loaf, 1032 kcals (4334 kJ), 11 g fat, of which 2 g saturated, 11 mg sodium (cuts into 12 or more slices, so less than 1 g fat per slice).

Per roll, 153 kcals (643 kJ), less than 2 g fat, of which saturated fat negligible, 2 mg sodium.

Method

1 Mix the flours and yeast in a bowl.

2 Add the oil and enough water to make a soft dough. Don't add all the water at once as you may not need it all – the amount of water required depends on the type of flour used. Add a little at a time until the mixture forms a ball, leaving the sides of the bowl clean. If the dough is too sticky, dust it with a bit of extra flour and mix it in.

3 Turn the dough out on to a floured surface and knead for about 10 minutes. Return it to the bowl and cover with cling film. Leave in a warm place for about 1–1¼ hours, or until the dough has risen roughly twice the size.

4 Grease either two 450-g (1-lb) loaf tins or a baking tray and set the oven to 230°C (450°F/gas mark 8). Then, knock the air out of the dough, turn it out on to a floured surface and knead for 5 minutes. Cut it in half and shape each to fit into the prepared tins

for loaves or make into round balls for rolls. Allow to rise for 45 to 60 minutes, until doubled in size. Brush the tops with a little milk before baking.

5 Bake for 25–30 minutes on the middle shelf for loaves or 12–15 minutes nearer the top for rolls. The bread is ready if the base sounds hollow when tapped. Turn out on to a wire tray. Both loaves and rolls freeze well.

Variation
Add 2 teaspoons of malt extract at step 2 to make a malt flavoured bread.

Sun-dried tomato and basil bread
Makes 2, yielding 16 slices

This is a tasty, focaccia-like bread to accompany soups or salads or just eat on its own. If you add sweet potato to the ingredients, this offers a tasty variation but the bread will be slightly heavier in texture. You can either enjoy this bread hot from the oven or leave it to cool and freeze it to use later as it freezes very well.

Tomatoes are rich in antioxidants, especially vitamins A and C. They also contain a substance called lycopene – one of the family of carotenoids – and there is evidence to suggest that this may have powerful anticarcinogenic properties. Lycopene is particularly highly concentrated in processed tomato products, such as ketchup, tinned tomatoes and tomato purée.

Sweet potatoes are the richest single food source of the antioxidant vitamins C, E and beta-carotene.

Ingredients

450 g (1 lb) strong white flour
1 heaped tsp dried basil
1 tsp fast-acting dried yeast
1 tsp paprika
1 tsp extra virgin olive oil
2 tsp tomato purée
170 ml (6 fl oz) water (200 ml/7 fl oz if not using sweet potato)

1 medium sweet potato (170 g/ 6 oz), peeled and boiled for 10 minutes until soft, then cut into small chunks
40 g ($1\frac{1}{2}$ oz) sun-dried tomatoes (dried weight)
extra flour for dusting

Nutritional analysis
Per slice, 122 kcals (512 kJ), 2 g fat, of which saturated fat negligible, 33 mg sodium.

Method

1 Mix together the flour, basil, yeast and paprika.
2 Add the olive oil, tomato purée, water and sweet potato, if using, and mix into a soft dough. If the dough is too sticky, add a little extra flour; if it is too dry, add a few more drops of water.
3 Turn the dough out on to a floured surface and knead for about 10 minutes. Return it to the bowl and cover with cling film. Allow to rise in a warm place for about 1–1½ hours, or until it has doubled in size.
4 Meanwhile, rehydrate the sun-dried tomatoes as directed on the packaging, which also removes salt used in drying them.
5 Knock the air out of the dough and place it on a floured surface. Knead briefly and then cut it into two. Roll each half into a round shape, roughly 20 cm (8 in) in diameter. Place the thin strips of sun-dried tomato on the dough so that both rounds are nicely covered. Knead in and roll the dough back into flat round shapes with a floured rolling pin. Score each round of dough into eighths with a knife (not quite cutting through).
6 Place on a greased baking tray and leave to rise in a warm place for about another hour or until it has doubled in size. Don't be tempted to start baking too soon. Towards the end of this time, preheat the oven to 220°C (425°F/gas mark 7).
7 Bake the bread in the preheated oven for 15–20 minutes. It is ready if the base sounds hollow when tapped. Turn out on to a wire cooling rack.

Chapattis
Makes 12

An excellent accompaniment to a spicy home-made curry (pages 93–4). Ideally they should be eaten immediately, but they do also freeze very well. Simply reheat them on the middle shelf of an oven preheated to 180°C (350°F/gas mark 4) for 10 minutes or pop them in a microwave set to high for about 10 seconds when you need them.

Ingredients

225 g (8 oz) plain wholemeal flour
150 ml ($\frac{1}{4}$ pint) cold water

extra flour for dusting
splash/spray light vegetable oil for greasing

Nutritional analysis

Per chapatti, 58 kcals (244 kJ), 0.5 g fat, of which saturated fat negligible, 0.6 mg sodium.

Method

1 Place the flour in a bowl and add sufficient water for the mixture to form a ball of soft dough, leaving the sides of the bowl clean. Sprinkle with a little more flour if the dough is too sticky or add a splash of water if it is too dry.
2 Transfer the dough to a floured surface and knead for about 10 minutes to get the gluten working – this makes the dough elastic. Cover with a damp tea towel or cling film and leave to rest for half an hour.
3 Prepare a frying pan or griddle, lightly brushing or spraying it with the oil.
4 Divide the dough into 12 small balls. Roll each ball flat on a floured surface with a rolling pin. Try to make them as thin as possible, but still oval shapes.
5 Heat up the griddle or frying pan to a medium heat (no added oil). Cook each chapatti on one side for about 1–2 minutes, until bubbles appear in the dough, then turn it over and cook the other side for the same length of time. (You might like to treat them like pancakes and toss them over.) Press them gently to expel the air before taking them from the griddle or pan and placing them on a warmed plate.

Pizza base
Makes 2 small or 1 large

To speed up making a pizza you can buy ready-made pizza bases, but you can also make your own very easily. You can make two or three at a time by doubling or tripling the recipe below and you'll find that they freeze very well. Just remove them from the freezer when you need them, defrost and use to make a pizza to your own special design (see the 'Meals in under 30 minutes' section later in the book).

You can use strong white flour, as in this recipe, to make a light, crispy base, or wholemeal flour for a more substantial base or a half-and-half mixture. Try out different combinations until you find the one that suits you.

If you intend to make lots of pizzas it's a good idea to invest in a circular pizza baking tray (the type with a few air holes in it, sometimes called a 'pizza crisper'). A tray 30 cm (12 in) in diameter will make a good-size base and you'll find that it's much easier to shape the dough into the round pizza shape than before because you can put the final touches to the shape when the dough is on the tray. You can stretch the dough and roll it to fit the shape, then push it right into the edge of the tray with your fingers. You can also freeze the pizza on the tray.

Ingredients
225 g (8 oz) strong white flour
1½ tsp fast-acting dried yeast
7–8 tbsp hand-hot water

1 tsp olive oil
extra flour for dusting

Nutritional analysis
Per large pizza base, 806 kcals (3385 kJ), 6 g fat, of which 1 g saturated, 10 mg sodium.

Method
1 Place the flour in a mixing bowl and stir in the dried yeast.
2 Add enough water, a tablespoon at a time, mixing to form a dough that makes a ball and leaves the sides of the bowl clean. The exact amount of water needed will depend on the flour used. If you use too much water, the dough will become very sticky, but don't despair. You can easily remedy this by sprinkling a little more flour into the bowl and mixing it in.

3 Transfer the dough to a flour-dusted surface and knead for 7–8 minutes. If you have an electric mixer with a dough hook this will shorten the time taken to knead the dough. Place it back in the bowl and coat the surface of the dough with the oil. Cover with a damp tea towel or cling film and leave to rise in a warm place for an hour or more until it has roughly doubled in size.

4 Grease a baking sheet or special pizza baking tray and preheat the oven to 220°C (425°F/gas mark 7). Remove the dough from the bowl and knead for 5 minutes on a floured surface. Then, roll it out into one or two round shapes using a rolling pin dusted with flour. Turn the dough frequently in a circular motion and stretch it with your fingers to form the shape. Place it on the prepared tray.

5 If the pizza base or bases is/are to be frozen, bake in the preheated oven for 5 minutes on the middle shelf. Otherwise, follow the Mushroom, red pepper and mozzarella pizza recipe (pages 156–7) for a tasty pizza.

Almond biscuits
Makes 12

Ingredients

85 g (3 oz) self-raising flour
25 g (1 oz) caster sugar
25 g (1 oz) oats
25 g (1 oz) flaked almonds
4 tsp rapeseed or light olive oil

1 egg
1 tbsp skimmed milk
1 tsp almond essence
1 glacé cherry, chopped into 12 small pieces

Nutritional analysis
Per biscuit, 70 kcals (294 kJ), 3 g fat, of which saturated fat negligible, 33 mg sodium.

Method

1 Grease a baking tray and preheat the oven to 180°C (350°F/gas mark 4). Sift together the flour and sugar into a mixing bowl, then mix in the oats and almonds.

2 Add the oil, egg, milk and almond essence. Mix together well until the mixture has a stiff, dropping consistency.

3 Spoon the mixture on to the prepared baking tray in 12 blobs

using 2 dessert spoons. Fill one spoon about half full with the mixture and then empty it on to the tray with the other. Slightly flatten and spread out each of the irregularly shaped blobs and, finally, add a small piece of glacé cherry to the centre of each for decoration.

4 Bake on the middle shelf of the preheated oven for about 15–20 minutes. Store in an airtight container or freeze.

Lemon biscuits
Makes 12

A variation on the Almond biscuits recipe.

Ingredients

85 g (3 oz) self-raising flour
25 g (1 oz) caster sugar
10 g ($\frac{1}{2}$ oz) oats
25 g (1 oz) flaked almonds
4 tsp rapeseed or light olive
   oil

1 egg
finely grated rind and 1 tbsp
   juice of 1 lemon
1 tsp honey
1 glacé cherry, chopped into
   12 small pieces

Nutritional analysis
Per biscuit, 78 kcals (328 kJ), 3 g fat, of which saturated fat negligible, 37 mg sodium.

Method
1 [as 1 on page 134]
2 Add the oil, egg, lemon rind and juice and honey. Mix together well until the mixture has a stiff, dropping consistency.
3 [as 3 above]
4 [as 4 above]

Chocolate and sultana cookies
Makes 12

Based on the Almond biscuits recipe, but chocolatey!

Ingredients
85 g (3 oz) self-raising flour
1 oz (25 g) drinking chocolate
10 g ($\frac{1}{2}$ oz) caster sugar
25 g (1 oz) oats
25 g (1 oz) sultanas

4 tsp rapeseed or light olive oil
1 egg
1 tbsp skimmed milk

Nutritional analysis
Each cookie provides 74 kcals (311 kJ), 2 g fat, of which saturated fat is negligible, 44 mg sodium.

Method
1 Grease a baking tray and preheat the oven to 180°C (350°F/gas mark 4). Sift together the flour, drinking chocolate and sugar into a mixing bowl, then mix in the oats and sultanas.
2 Add the oil, egg and milk. Mix together until the mixture has a stiff, dropping consistency.
3 [as 3 on pages 134–5, minus cherry]
4 [as 4 on page 135]

Currant and red wine biscuits
Makes 24

This recipe and the next are part of the original selection in the companion volume *How to Keep Your Cholesterol in Check*. These recipes continue to be a popular choice with readers. They are easy to make, low in fat and full of healthy, cholesterol-lowering ingredients.

Ingredients
115 g (4 oz) wholemeal flour
50 g (2 oz) oats
2 tsp cinnamon
25 g (1 oz) flaked almonds
2 tbsp (30 ml) olive or rapeseed oil

3 tbsp freshly squeezed (or from a carton) orange juice
2 tbsp red wine or red grape juice if preferred
115 g (4 oz) currants
extra flour for dusting

Nutritional analysis
Per biscuit, 55 kcals (231 kJ), 2 g fat, of which saturated fat negligible, 1 mg sodium.

Method
1 Grease a baking tray and preheat the oven to 190°C (375°F/gas mark 5). Mix the flour, oats, cinnamon and almonds together in a food processor or mixer.
2 Add the oil, orange juice and red wine or red grape juice.
3 Mix together until the mixture can be formed into a ball (add a little extra juice if necessary).
4 Add the currants and mix them in briefly.
5 Place on a floured surface and roll out thinly with a rolling pin.
6 Cut into about 24 round biscuit shapes with a 6.5-cm (2½-in) diameter cutter.
7 Using a palette knife, transfer the biscuits to the prepared baking tray and bake in the preheated oven for about 15 minutes on the middle shelf. Transfer to a cooling rack, then either store in an airtight container or freeze.

Fruity oat bran buns
Makes 15

Oat bran has distinct heart-health benefits. It has been shown to have a cholesterol-lowering effect and, in a number of studies, beneficial effects have been demonstrated for a daily intake of around 50 g (2 oz). Three of these buns will provide this amount of oat bran. You can also try sprinkling oat bran on your cereal or adding it to soups, stews or casseroles or else use it to make a delicious porridge.

Ingredients
250 g (9 oz) oat bran
1 tbsp baking powder
25 g (1 oz) soft brown sugar
1½ tsp ground cinnamon
1 tsp mixed spice
25 g (1 oz) chopped walnuts

½ eating apple, peeled and grated
1 tbsp light olive oil
350 ml (12 fl oz) semi-skimmed or soya milk
85 g (3 oz) mixed fruit

Nutritional analysis
Per bun, 109 kcals (458 kJ), 4 g fat, of which 1 g saturated, 25 mg sodium, and eating 3 provides beneficial intake of 50 g (2 oz) oat bran.

Method
1 Grease one or more bun trays sufficient to make 15 buns. Preheat the oven to 220°C (425°F/gas mark 7).
2 Blend together the oat bran, baking powder, sugar, spices and nuts in a food processor or mixing bowl.
3 Add the apple, olive oil and milk and mix together. Allow the liquid to soak in for 1–2 minutes.
4 Add the mixed fruit and give it a final short mix without chopping the fruit too much.
5 Spoon into the prepared bun tins, making 15 even-sized buns. Bake in the preheated oven for about 15 minutes.
6 Leave for a short time, then turn out on to a cooling rack. They keep best in a plastic container or bag in the fridge or can be frozen. They can be warmed up, from frozen, by placing them in a microwave and cooking on high for about 40 seconds per bun.

Carrot and orange cake slices
Makes 12

Carrots are high in beta-carotene – an important antioxidant. It may seem a bit odd to use them in cake slices (or even a Christmas pudding as we do on pages 118–19), but their nutritious content and sweet taste make them a valuable ingredient. Mrs Beeton, the famous Victorian cooking authority, even encouraged their use in jams!

Ingredients

170 g (6 oz) self-raising flour

40 g (1½ oz) caster sugar

2 level tsp baking powder

2 tsp honey

zest of ½ large orange

1 tbsp orange juice

1 (85-g/3-oz) carrot, finely grated

50 g (2 oz) unsaturated margarine

1 tbsp rapeseed oil

4 tbsp skimmed milk

1 egg

Nutritional analysis
Per slice, 118 kcals (496 kJ), 5 g fat, of which 1 g saturated, 170 mg sodium.

Method
1 Mix together the flour, sugar and baking powder in a food processor or mixer.
2 Add the honey, orange zest and juice, carrot (reserving a third of it), margarine, oil, milk and egg. Beat for about 1 minute in the food processor or 2 minutes at high speed in a mixer.
3 Transfer the mixture into the prepared cake tin using a spoon or spatula. Level the top and sprinkle the reserved carrot evenly over the mixture.
4 Bake on the middle shelf of the preheated oven for 25–30 minutes.
5 Allow to cool for 5 minutes, then cut into 12 slices.

Raisin malt loaf
Makes 14 slices

A perennial favourite from the companion volume *How to Keep Your Cholesterol in Check*.

Walnuts provide the body with essential omega-3 fatty acids, which are beneficial for the heart (see Chapter 2). Raisins and tea are rich in flavonoids, which are potent antioxidants. Altogether, this loaf has some powerful heart-protecting ingredients.

Ingredients

285 g (10 oz) seedless raisins
40 g (1½ oz) soft light brown sugar
2 tbsp malt extract
275 ml (½ pint) hot tea
400 g (14 oz) self-raising wholemeal flour
50 g (2 oz) chopped walnuts
1 egg
8 tbsp skimmed milk

Nutritional analysis
Raisin malt loaf per slice, 195 kcals (819 kJ), 4 g fat, of which saturated fat negligible, 25 mg sodium.

Method
1 Place the raisins, sugar, malt extract and hot tea in a bowl. Stir and leave to soak overnight.
2 Grease a 900-g (2-lb) loaf tin and preheat the oven to 170°C (325°F/gas mark 3). Then, once the fruit has soaked, add the flour, walnuts, egg and milk to it and mix together well.
3 Transfer the mixture to the prepared loaf tin and bake in the middle of the preheated oven for 45 minutes. Then, turn the oven down to 150°C (300°F/gas mark 2) and bake for a further 15–20 minutes, or until a skewer inserted into the centre of the loaf comes out clean. Leave to cool in the tin for a few minutes, then turn out on to a cooling rack to finish cooling down. Slice and enjoy.

Sultana, date and walnut loaf

Dates are an excellent source of cholesterol-lowering soluble fibre and are full of antioxidant vitamins.

Ingredients

170 g (6 oz) sultanas	115 g (4 oz) ready-to-eat dates,
25 g (1 oz) soft light brown	cut into raisin-sized chunks
sugar	225 g (8 oz) cooking apples,
150 ml ($\frac{1}{4}$ pint) hot tea	cored, peeled and chopped
400 g (14 oz) self-raising	as dates
wholemeal flour	1 egg
50 g (2 oz) chopped walnuts	8 tbsp skimmed milk

Nutritional analysis
Sultana, date and walnut loaf per slice, 190 kcals (798 kJ), 4 g fat, of which saturated fat negligible, 15 mg sodium.

Method
1 Place the sultanas, sugar and hot tea in a bowl. Stir and leave to soak overnight.
2 Grease a 900-g (2-lb) loaf tin and preheat the oven to 170°C (325°F/gas mark 3). Then, once the fruit has soaked, add the flour, walnuts, dates, apple, egg and milk to it and mix together well.
3 [as 3 above]

Oaty crunch bars
Makes 16

Another old favourite from the companion volume *How to Keep Your Cholesterol in Check*.

Studies in Canada have shown that a diet low in saturated fat and rich in foods such as oats, plant sterols, soya proteins and nuts can reduce cholesterol dramatically. This 'Portfolio' diet on its own has even produced results rivalling the cholesterol-lowering effects of drugs such as the first-generation statins taken alongside standard low-fat regimes.

If you can't find the larger jumbo oats, just replace with ordinary rolled oats.

Ingredients

1 tbsp malt extract	85 g (3 oz) jumbo oats
2 tbsp rapeseed oil	140 g (5 oz) rolled oats
75 g (2½ oz) low-fat	50 g (2 oz) sultanas
unsaturated margarine	honey, for brushing top
1 tbsp golden syrup	1 tbsp sesame seeds

Nutritional analysis
Per bar, 108 kcals (454 kJ), 5 g fat, of which 1 g saturated, 41 mg sodium.

Method
1 Grease the base of a 28 × 18-cm (11 × 7-in) shallow cake tin and preheat the oven to 180°C (350°F/gas mark 4). Then, place the malt extract, oil, margarine and golden syrup in a large saucepan. Stir and heat gently for about 1 minute, until the margarine has just melted.
2 Add the oats and sultanas, mixing them in thoroughly. Then press the mixture into the prepared tin and smooth down the top. Mark out 16 slices using a knife and press back any oats disturbed by the cutting.
3 Brush the honey over the top, then sprinkle the sesame seeds over and press down into the mixture, taking care not to disturb the cut edges. Bake in the preheated oven for 20 minutes. Cool for at least 1 hour before removing the bars from the tin. Store in an airtight container or freeze.

Fruit scones
Makes approximately 20

The main secret to making excellent scones is to ensure that when you roll out the dough, it isn't too thin. It needs to be about 2-cm ($\frac{3}{4}$-in) thick. Serve with a plant sterol or stanol spread or an unsaturated margarine, thinly spread with plum jam (page 73). Delicious!

Ingredients

450 (1 lb) self-raising flour
2 level tsp baking powder
85 g (3 oz) unsaturated
  margarine

275 ml ($\frac{1}{2}$ pint) semi-skimmed
  or soya milk
115 g (4 oz) sultanas
extra flour for dusting

Nutritional analysis
Per scone, 130 kcals (546 kJ), 4 g fat, of which 1 g saturated, 166 mg sodium.

Method
1 Lightly grease a baking tray and preheat the oven to 220°C (425°F/gas mark 7). Then sift together the flour and baking powder into a bowl. Mix in the margarine until the mixture resembles breadcrumbs. Then add the milk slowly, a little at a time. Mix it in lightly and use just enough to make a soft – not sticky – dough. Then add the sultanas, making sure that they are well distributed in the mixture.
2 Turn the dough out on to a floured surface and roll out to a thickness of about 2 cm ($\frac{3}{4}$ in). Use a 6.5-cm ($2\frac{1}{2}$-in) cutter to cut out the scones.
3 Place the scones on the prepared baking tray and sprinkle a little flour over them. Bake them in the preheated oven for about 12 minutes, or until they have browned slightly on top. Transfer to a cooling rack, then either store in an airtight container or freeze.

Grandma's favourite fruit cake
Makes 12–14 slices

The secret of this delicious cake lies in soaking the fruit overnight.

Ingredients

200 g (7 oz) mixed dried fruit, including peel
40g (1½ oz) ready-to-eat dried apricots, finely chopped
25 g (1 oz) glacé cherries, sliced into eighths
2 rounded tsp mixed spice
1 tsp soft brown sugar
1 tbsp dry sherry or orange juice

200 ml (⅓ pint) hot tea
115 g (4 oz) wholemeal self-raising flour
115 g (4 oz) white self-raising flour
1 level tsp baking powder
100 g (3½ oz) low-fat unsaturated margarine
2 eggs
handful flaked almonds

Nutritional analysis

Per slice, 162 kcals (680 kJ), 5 g fat, of which 1 g saturated, 171 mg sodium.

Method

1 Mix together the fruit, reserving 8 pieces of cherry, the mixed spice, sugar and sherry in a bowl and pour the hot tea over them. Stir and leave to soak overnight.
2 Grease and line an 18-cm (7-in) cake tin and preheat the oven to 170°C (325°F/gas mark 3). Sift the flours and baking powder into a mixing bowl, lightly mix together and then add the margarine, eggs and soaked fruit mixture. Mix well before transferring to the prepared cake tin. Spread the flaked almonds over the top and decorate with the reserved cherry pieces.
3 Bake in the middle of the preheated oven for 1 hour. Then, turn it down to 150°C (300°F/gas mark 2) and bake for a further 10 minutes or until a skewer inserted into the cake comes out clean. Leave to cool in the tin, then turn it out on to a wire cooling rack. Store in an airtight container.

Variation

For a very low-fat cake (just over 1 g per slice), replace the margarine and chopped apricots with a prune or apricot purée made using 115 g (4 oz) ready-to-eat prunes or apricots and 1 tbsp water.

Mince pies
Makes 10

Here is an easy recipe for making mince pies, using the Mincemeat recipe given on page 75 to provide the filling.

One of the secrets of certain types of bowling in cricket is for the batsman to use a 'soft hands' technique and the same goes for making pastry! Treat the ingredients gently and try to keep your hands as soft and cool as possible. Also, don't despair if you seem to be running out of pastry at the rolling stage. Just collect up the odd bits and pieces, form a new ball from them and roll out again. It's amazing how many rounds you can still make from the leftovers.

When you're making mince pies for Christmas or for any other party occasion, bake in bulk. Double up or even treble the recipe, baking 20 or 30 mince pies all in one go. They will freeze beautifully, so you can be prepared for the festivities well in advance. You can use the leftover egg whites to make Meringues (page 114).

Ingredients

85 g (3 oz) plain flour
50 g (2 oz) self-raising flour
25 g (1 oz) cornflour
1 rounded tsp caster sugar
75 g (2½ oz) low-fat
    unsaturated soft margarine
    (put it in the freezer until
    cold and firm)

1 egg yolk mixed with 1 tsp
    cold water
extra flour, for dusting
200 g (7 oz) Mincemeat (page
    74)
a little skimmed milk, for
    brushing pastry

Nutritional analysis
Per mince pie, 178 kcals (748 kJ), 4 g fat, of which 1 g saturated, 77 mg sodium.

Method
1 Sift the flours, cornflour and sugar into a food processor or mixing bowl. Be flamboyant – hold the sieve up high and tap its sides so the flour aerates as it descends into the mixing bowl below.
2 Add the margarine and whizz in the processor for a few seconds, until the mixture resembles breadcrumbs. Then add the egg yolk and water mixture. Whizz round briefly again, in pulses, until the

whole mixture forms into larger breadcrumbs. Then gently form the mixture into a ball using your hands. Add a few extra drops of water if necessary, but the less water you use, the better the pastry. Place the pastry in a polythene bag in the fridge and leave to rest for 30 minutes.

3 Grease a bun tin or tins (so you can make 10 mince pies) and preheat the oven to 190°C (375°F/gas mark 5). Then place the dough on a surface dusted with flour. Using a rolling pin, roll out two-thirds of the pastry quite thinly, then cut it into 10 rounds with a 7.5-cm (3-in) fluted cutter. Do the same with the remaining third, this time using a 6.5-cm (2½-in) cutter.

4 Place the larger rounds in the prepared bun tin. Fill each with about 1 heaped tsp Mincemeat. Brush the top edges of the pastry with the milk and carefully place the smaller rounds on top of the Mincemeat to form a pastry lid. Seal by pinching the edges of the pastry together. Make 2–3 snips in the top of each pastry lid and brush the lids with milk. Bake on the middle shelf of the preheated oven for 20 minutes.

Drinks

Before we look at individual drinks, we should perhaps first of all dispel one widely held myth about the amount of water we need to drink: that we need to drink at least eight glasses of water a day, equivalent to about 2 litres ($3\frac{1}{2}$ pints). Many people have found that's a lot to drink in one day! Well, don't worry. The claim that we need to drink this amount of plain water each day is just not true. The idea probably came from the misinterpretation of a recommendation by the US Food and Nutrition Board in the 1980s that we should drink about 1 ml of water for every calorie of food consumed, so, for a 2000 calorie intake, that's 2 litres ($3\frac{1}{2}$ pints). However, people forgot to read the next part of the report, which made clear that we already get quite a lot of this fluid from prepared foods. It's important to have a good intake of fluids, to prevent dehydration, kidney problems and constipation, for example, and water is an important fluid source. However, we can take fluids in all sorts of forms. Research from the Center for Human Nutrition in Omaha, Nebraska, in the USA, has shown that water in tea, coffee and soft drinks counts just as well towards our intake of fluids as plain water,

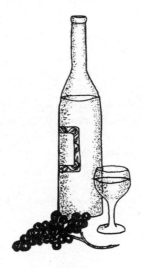

but, this said, it's not good to have too high an intake of caffeine or sugary drinks. We also obtain fluids from many other sources, such as milk, and fruit and vegetables. In fact, about a third of an adult's daily fluid intake comes from what we eat rather than what we drink.

It's certainly a good idea to drink plenty of fluids, including plain water, but you don't need to force water down you like some sort of cleansing medicine! Plain water provides a good, low-calorie drink; it's good for you and drinking 2 litres ($3\frac{1}{2}$ pints) a day isn't going to do you any harm, but drinking that much plain water is not a necessary requirement for healthy living. If you tend to get easily dehydrated (signs are headaches, irritation, bad breath, dark urine, constipation and low energy), just increase your intake of fluids and, if you're imbibing a dehydrating drink, such as wine, then drink a similar amount of water alongside it. Otherwise, relax and enjoy the range of healthy drinks on offer.

Fresh fruit pressé

This is just a fancy way to introduce different ideas about squeezing fruits! If you have a blender, you can make all kinds of exciting drinks – and no added sugar is required.

- Try freshly squeezed orange juice as a delightful start to the day.
- Try peaches, mangoes or strawberries for deliciously flavoursome drinks.
- If you find that grapefruit juice is a bit bitter for your taste, try adding some banana to it in the blender.
- Add other things, such as passion fruit, or mix in some ready prepared juice from a carton to give a sweeter flavour to your blended fruit. Both mangoes and strawberries, for example, combine very well with orange juice, while passion fruit brings out the flavour of strawberries. Apple juice, bananas and strawberries also make a delicious combination.
- If you want a nice cool drink on a summer's day, just add a few ice cubes to the blender along with the fruit or make ice lollies by freezing juice in special plastic ice lolly containers.
- Turn your drink into a sumptuous fool by adding some custard (see recipes on pages 123–4) or make a refreshing sorbet (pages 121–3) or smoothie, like our Strawberry smoothie (page 148).

- You don't always need to squeeze the juice out of the fruit to make a delicious drink. Try adding a couple of slices of orange, lemon or lime to iced water or sparkling mineral water for a refreshing lunchtime drink.

Strawberry smoothie
Makes 4 wine glass-sized drinks

Smoothies are rich, creamy drinks that can be made using all sorts of fruit in a blender or food processor. Try your own special blends.

Ingredients
10 tbsp low-fat bio yogurt with
  a little soya milk if you
  prefer it less thick
200 g (7 oz) strawberries
2 passion fruits, pulp only,
  sieved to remove seeds
2 tsp honey

Nutritional analysis
Per glass, 104 kcals (437 kJ), 1 g fat, of which 0.5 g saturates, 110 mg sodium.

Method
1 Just whizz the ingredients round in a blender or food processor and pour out your smoothie into the wine glass.

Non-alcoholic tropical fruit punch
Makes approximately 26 small wine glass-sized drinks
To make smaller quantities just reduce the ingredients proportionally.

We have used a blend of orange, pineapple, apple and passion fruit juices, with banana and mango purée, but all sorts of blends will work. Just choose your own favourite pure tropical fruit juice carton (preferably one with around 10 g sugar per 100 ml or less).

Ingredients

750 ml (1¼ pints) soda water
250 ml (½ pint) dry ginger ale
2 × 1-litre (1¾-pint) cartons
  tropical fruit juice
1 large orange, thinly sliced,
  pips removed, slices halved

½ lemon, thinly sliced, pips
  removed
250 ml (½ pint) cold water
1 level tsp mixed spice
pinch ground nutmeg
ice cubes, to serve

Nutritional analysis
Per glass, 30 kcals (126 kJ), fat negligible, of which saturated fat negligible, sodium negligible.

Method
1 Put the bottles of soda water and dry ginger ale in the fridge to cool, ready to add to the punch later.
2 When ready, place all the ingredients apart from the soda water and ginger ale in a large punch bowl – any serving bowl of 3-litre (just over 5-pint) capacity will do. Stir and chill in the fridge for about 2 hours.
3 Pour in the measured amounts of soda water and ginger ale and stir in the ice cubes.

Tea and coffee

You can enjoy both tea and coffee without apologizing to your body for drinking them. They both contain caffeine – as do other drinks, such as cocoa, drinking chocolate and cola – which has a stimulating effect on the heart and central nervous system, but this isn't necessarily a bad thing. On the whole, caffeine only really causes problems when we have too much of it. Then, it can become mildly addictive, result in palpitations and difficulty in sleeping. In moderation, caffeine is a relatively harmless substance and there's certainly no good evidence to suggest that it causes heart disease.

As far as tea is concerned, there's a good deal of favourable research showing that drinking tea can have a lipid-lowering effect. It's full of flavonoids and phenols, which have potent antioxidant properties, and there is also some suggestion that it might help to thin the blood and boost the immune system. Most research studies examining the link between tea consumption and heart disease indicate that drinking two or more cups a day probably actually has a *protective* effect on the heart. So, you can enjoy your regular cuppa and develop your taste for teas of all types. If you normally stick to the usual brown or Indian tea, why not try some fruit-flavoured teas or see how you get on with the distinctive flavours of Earl Grey or darjeeling tea – sometimes known as the 'queen of teas'?

As for coffee, the main point to consider is the way in which it is brewed. If you allow the coffee grounds to soak in boiling water (as in the cafetière method) or repeatedly boil the grounds, as in the Scandinavian approach, this can have a cholesterol-raising effect. If instead you use filter papers, these tend to remove the cholesterol-raising substance from the coffee grounds, and instant coffee lacks this substance. In fact, in one piece of research, it was found that people who drank coffee regularly – mainly *instant* coffee drinkers in this particular study – tended to have less heart disease than those who drank little or no coffee. If the caffeine is a problem, there are some excellent brands of decaffeinated coffee available. They won't reduce the brewing-related cholesterol effects but they will reduce the palpitations and insomnia.

So, there's no reason to avoid coffee for the sake of good heart health. It could even be doing some good. However, if you need to keep a fairly close eye on your cholesterol levels, it would be sensible to opt for filter or instant coffee as your *regular* method of making coffee, keeping any other methods you like to use for special treats.

Beware drinks with lots of added sugar

Too much sugary fizz (or 'liquid candy' as some carbonated soft drinks have been called) can be a major danger to heart health. On the whole, it's best to choose drinks based on fruit juices rather than sugary fizz and even these should be drunk only in moderation (see page 23).

In America, carbonated drinks constitute the single biggest source of added, refined sugars in the diet and lots of sugar means lots of calories. The consumption of such drinks has increased massively in recent years, as has the size of the individual can of drink and also the size of the individuals who drink them!

The World Health Organization has expressed serious concern about the increased consumption of sugar-sweetened drinks, especially by children. It is suggested that each additional can or glass of sugar-dense drink that a child drinks each day will increase the risk of becoming obese by 60 per cent and, as we know, obesity is inextricably linked to diabetes and heart disease.

Milk

Milk is an important source of nutrients – especially protein, calcium, and a wide range of vitamins and minerals. However, as full-fat milk contains more saturated fat than skimmed or semi-skimmed milk, we suggest using the reduced-fat varieties for a heart-healthy diet. These lower-fat milks are still excellent sources of calcium, which is especially important for the prevention of osteoporosis – a disease leading to thinned and easily broken bones.

Drink milk on its own or in cocoa or drinking chocolate or with breakfast cereals or use to make custard or rice pudding.

You can try soya milk as a variation. It has a similar fat content to semi-skimmed milk, but the composition of the fat is slightly different – it contains a little less saturated fat, a little more polyunsaturated fat and is a source of important omega-3 fatty acids. In addition, the soya protein content of the milk helps to keep cholesterol levels in check. However, unlike ordinary milk, soya milk is low in calcium, so it's useful to choose varieties fortified with calcium and vitamins where possible.

Mulled wine
Makes approximately 25 small wine glass-sized drinks

Alcoholic drinks have been discussed earlier (at the end of Chapter 4), but we include here one delicious recipe for mulled wine. It makes a wonderful warming drink for a cold winter's night, especially around Christmas and New Year. It is also an excellent party drink at any time of year.

To make smaller quantities for a smaller number of people, simply halve the amounts in the recipe, but keep the half an orange, and use three cloves instead of five.

In medieval times, 'mulled' – that is, heated and spiced up – wines were known as Ypocras or Hipocris, after the physician Hippocrates, of 'Hippocratic oath' fame. The drink was considered to be very healthy and, in comparison to the frequently putrid drinking water at the time, it certainly would have been. It's also possible, though, that this view of mulled wine as a healthy drink was an early recognition of what we now know to be the potent antioxidant properties of wine (see Chapter 3).

Ingredients

1 litre (1$\frac{3}{4}$ pints) orange juice
$\frac{1}{2}$ orange, well washed, with 5 cloves pushed into the peel
$\frac{1}{2}$ tsp ground ginger
pinch ground nutmeg
2 cinnamon sticks
170 g (6 oz) soft brown sugar

1 large orange, washed and thinly sliced, pips removed
1 unwaxed lemon, prepared as orange
3 × 75-cl bottles red wine (it doesn't need to be expensive)

Nutritional analysis

Per glass, 114 kcals (479 kJ), fat negligible, of which saturated fat negligible, 10 mg sodium.

Method

1 Place the orange juice, half orange stuck with cloves, ginger, nutmeg and cinnamon sticks in a pan large enough to take 3 litres (just over 5 pints) mulled wine, such as a preserving pan. Add the sugar and bring the contents to the boil, stirring frequently until the sugar has dissolved.

2 Remove the pan from the heat, add the slices of orange and lemon and leave to stand for 10 minutes.

3 Pour in the wine and heat, but do not allow to boil as this tends to spoil the flavour of the blend of wine and spices. Set over a very low heat for $\frac{1}{2}$ to 1 hour to allow the flavours to blend. Then serve in warmed wine glasses.

4 When the flavours have blended nicely, you can take the pan off the heat and, instead of heating the whole contents of the pan, simply ladle some into a glass and heat for 30 seconds or so in the microwave. Check frequently to make sure that the liquid doesn't come to the boil.

5 If you make too much mulled wine for one evening, bottle the liquid (not the fruit, which tends to go bitter) or transfer it to a jug and heat up a glassful at a time the next day.

Meals in under 30 minutes

Spicy egg scramblette
Serves 2

This is a hybrid recipe – something between scrambled egg and an omelette, so we've had to make our own name for it and we came up with egg scramblette!

It uses just one egg between two people. Although eggs are a source of protein and vitamins, the yolks contain both saturated fat and cholesterol. This is not the case with egg whites, though, which are fine. On the plus side, the type of cholesterol in eggs and other foods – so-called 'dietary cholesterol' – doesn't have too much impact on our blood cholesterol levels (see Chapter 1), so eggs aren't all bad.

Interestingly, some people appear to have an 'egg-eating gene' that allows them to eat a large amount of eggs without any apparent adverse effects on their blood lipid levels. For practical purposes, though, it's probably best to assume that you don't have this gene and, if you have been advised to watch your cholesterol levels, we suggest keeping to a maximum of three to four eggs a week and, for people with FH (page 2), no more than two eggs. For extra benefit, try using eggs enriched with omega-3.

Ingredients

115 g (4 oz) broccoli florets or same quantity fresh spinach, stems trimmed off
1 egg
90 ml (3 fl oz) skimmed milk
$\frac{1}{2}$ tsp turmeric
1 tsp rapeseed oil
1 shallot, finely chopped
1 small potato, finely chopped

$\frac{1}{4}$ red pepper, deseeded and sliced
1 garlic clove, crushed or finely chopped
50 g (2 oz) mushrooms, sliced
$\frac{1}{2}$ tsp paprika
2 pinches mixed herbs
freshly ground black pepper
1 tomato, sliced

Nutritional analysis
Per serving, 130 kcals (546 kJ), 6 g fat, of which 1 g saturated, 78 mg sodium.

For ham variation, 153 kcals (643 kJ), 6 g fat, of which 1 g saturated, 377 mg sodium.

Method
1 Steam the broccoli florets for 6–7 minutes, until tender or cook the spinach in a saucepan with 2 tsp water for 4–5 minutes over a low heat. Strain, cover and set to one side.
2 Mix the egg and milk in a jug. Add the turmeric and mix to a smooth liquid.
3 Place the oil in a large frying pan and heat. Add the shallot, potato and red pepper. Cover and cook for about 3 minutes over a gentle heat. Stir occasionally or just shake the pan to avoid the vegetables sticking and burning.
4 Add the garlic, mushrooms and paprika. Cover and cook for a further 4 minutes. Stir from time to time to prevent burning. Meanwhile, slice the broccoli florets in half or cut the spinach with scissors and then add to the pan. Sprinkle the mixed herbs over the top, stir and cook for about 1 minute.
5 Give the egg mix a final stir in the jug, season well with pepper, then pour into the pan. Move the vegetables around to coat them with the egg mix. Cook for about 2–3 minutes, stirring from time to time until the liquid ceases to be runny and the egg is well set.
6 Spoon out on to warm plates. Decorate with the tomato slices and serve with a piece of toast and side salad. You may also enjoy a dash of lycopene-rich tomato ketchup.

Variation
Use chopped ham instead of mushrooms, adding it in step 4.

Lentil and tomato soup
Serves 4

We suggest that you make double the quantity of the home-made Vegetable stock recipe (pages 104–5), so you always have some for soups and other meals. If you use stock cubes, it is best to use half a stock cube to 275 ml ($\frac{1}{2}$ pint) of water to adjust for the fact that they tend to be high in salt.

This soup is delicious served piping hot with warm wholemeal bread or Sun-dried tomato and basil bread (pages 130–1).

Ingredients
1 tbsp olive oil
1 medium onion, finely
  chopped
1 garlic clove, crushed
115 g (4 oz) dried red lentils

1 × 400-g (14-oz) tin chopped
  tomatoes
850 ml (1$\frac{1}{2}$ pints) Vegetable
  stock
1 tsp dried thyme

Nutritional analysis
Per serving, 138 kcals (580 kJ), 2 g fat, of which saturated fat negligible, 470 mg sodium.

Method
1 Heat the oil in a large saucepan. Add the onion and garlic and fry together over a low heat for about 5–6 minutes, until they have softened.
2 Rinse and drain the lentils, then stir them into the pan, followed by the tomatoes. Add the Vegetable stock and thyme. Bring to the boil, then simmer gently for about 20 minutes, or until the lentils have softened.
3 Put half the soup in a liquidizer (leaving the other half out gives the soup a nice, chunky texture). Then return the liquidized soup to the saucepan, heat and serve.

Mushroom, red pepper and mozzarella pizza with pine nuts and olives
Serves 4

Once you have made your own Pizza base (pages 133–4) or bought a ready-made one, you're all set to enjoy a wonderful light meal in under 30 minutes! Try a variety of ingredients for toppings – roasted butternut squash is particularly nice, but takes a bit more time in preparation. If you need to reduce the fat, just put on less mozzarella cheese or leave it out altogether.

Ingredients

1 × pizza base
1 × 400-g (14-oz) tin chopped tomatoes
1 garlic clove
2 tsp tomato ketchup
freshly ground black pepper
115 g (4 oz) mushrooms, finely sliced

half red pepper, deseeded and sliced into thin strips
3 olives, halved
50 g (2 oz) grated mozzarella cheese
10 g ($\frac{1}{2}$ oz) pine nuts
2 tsp olive oil

Nutritional analysis

Pizza topping, per serving, 95 kcals (399 kJ), 6 g fat, of which 2 g saturated, 234 mg sodium.

Pizza topping plus base, per serving, 296 kcals (1243 kJ), 7 g fat, of which 2 g saturated, 232 mg sodium.

A ready-made 150-g ($5\frac{1}{2}$-oz) pizza base will tend to add a little extra fat and sodium (usually about 0.75 g fat and 125 mg sodium per serving) to the ingredients of the fully home-made pizza.

Method

1 Prepare the pizza base.
2 Preheat the oven to 220°C (425°F/gas mark 7), then prepare the topping by pouring the tinned tomatoes and crushed garlic clove into a saucepan. Bring to the boil, uncovered, then cook over a medium heat for 15 minutes, until the contents have cooked down to make a nice sauce. Stir occasionally to prevent burning.
3 Add the tomato ketchup to the sauce and season with black pepper. Spread the sauce evenly over the pizza base. (If you like a smoother topping, you can whizz the mixture for a couple of seconds in a food processor before spreading.)

4 Place the slices of mushroom round the edge and centre of the base. Add the strips of red pepper, together with the olive halves. Sprinkle the cheese over the pizza and top with the pine nuts.
5 Finally, drizzle the oil over the pizza. If you are using a defrosted semi-baked pizza base, place it directly on the top oven shelf with a baking tray on the shelf below to collect any drips. Otherwise, place your finished pizza on an oiled baking tray or special pizza crisper tray. Bake in the preheated oven for 10–12 minutes, until the cheese has melted and is slightly golden in places. Cut into quarters and serve with a side salad.

Spaghetti bolognese – the quick version
Serves 4

This is a quicker version of the recipe on pages 99–100, using a jar of a tomato pasta sauce. There are lots of very healthy sauces, some organic, using ingredients such as extra virgin olive oil, but still keeping the fat content low – around 2 per cent, for example. A jar can replace quite a few of the ingredients in the fuller recipe and it will save about an hour in preparation time.

Ingredients

2 tsp extra virgin olive oil
1 medium onion, finely chopped
1 garlic clove, crushed or finely chopped
225 g (8 oz) Quorn mince

1 × 450-g (1-lb) jar tomato pasta sauce
freshly ground black pepper
225–340 g 8–12 oz) spaghetti
2 tsp finely grated Parmesan cheese

Nutritional analysis
Per serving, 373 kcals (1567 kJ), 8 g fat, of which 1 g saturated, 767 mg sodium.

Method
1 Place the oil in a large flameproof casserole or frying pan. Add the onion and cook over a gentle heat for 5–6 minutes.
2 Add the garlic and Quorn mince and fry for about 3 minutes.
3 Add the jar of tomato sauce, bring to the boil, then simmer for 10 minutes. Season to taste with black pepper.

4 While the sauce is cooking, place the spaghetti in a pan of boiling water and cook for about the same length of time (or according to the instructions on the pack).
5 Drain the spaghetti and serve. Spoon the bolognese sauce on top and sprinkle a little Parmesan cheese over each serving.

Pasta with pesto and mushrooms
Serves 4

This recipe includes pine nuts and walnuts, so it is not especially low in fat. However, these fats are of the good variety – mostly mono- and polyunsaturated fats, the sort that have beneficial effects on heart health.

An easy way to judge the amount of pasta required is to half fill the bowl in which one person's cooked pasta is to be served with dry pasta. This will then be just about the right amount for one person. So, for four people, you can fill two bowls with the dry pasta and this should be sufficient, when cooked, for four servings.

Ingredients

quick-cook pasta sufficient for 4 people (see above)
1 tsp extra virgin olive oil
1 garlic clove, crushed or finely chopped
225 g (8 oz) mushrooms, sliced
8 tsp low-fat (16 per cent) pesto sauce
25 g (1 oz) walnuts, roughly chopped
2 tbsps low-fat yogurt
2 large tomatoes, sliced
handful fresh basil leaves, chopped

Nutritional analysis
Per serving, 365 kcals (1533 kJ), 10 g fat, of which 2 g saturated, 54 mg sodium.

Method
1 Place the pasta in a large saucepan with boiling water and cook for 10–12 minutes, or according to instructions.
2 While the pasta is cooking, heat the oil in another large saucepan, add the garlic and mushrooms and fry over a very low heat for about 5–6 minutes, stirring frequently or shaking the pan to prevent burning.

3 Stir in the pesto sauce and walnuts and heat for a further 2 minutes. Remove the pan from the heat.

4 When the pasta has cooked, drain it and stir into the mushrooms and pesto sauce. Cook over a low heat for a further 2 minutes, stirring continuously. Add the yogurt, a little at a time, during the last minute.

5 Spoon into serving bowls, decorate with the tomato slices and sprinkle the fresh basil leaves over. Try a little Mango chutney (pages 70–1) with it as a tasty accompaniment.

Quick meals using pre-prepared Ratatouille

These quick meal suggestions are based on the use of portions of previously prepared Ratatouille (pages 96–7). However, as the Ratatouille doesn't take much more than half an hour to prepare, you could also make it from scratch if you had just over 30 minutes to spare.

Tortillas or Pancakes with Ratatouille

Fill tortillas or Pancakes (pages 162–3) with the Ratatouille and serve with salad and a spoonful of yogurt. You can prepare the Pancakes in batches and freeze. They and the tortillas can be heated up in a minute or so in a microwave or a few minutes longer in the oven.

Cheat's curry

Add a spoonful or more of curry paste, according to taste, to the Ratatouille and heat up the mixture in a saucepan. Serve on a bed of rice. As accompaniments you could try a dressing-free tomato and lettuce salad, or diced cucumber in yogurt, dusted with paprika (a cucumber raita), or slices of banana or Mango chutney (pages 70–1) with chapattis or poppadoms. We have included a recipe for Chapattis (page 132). These are suitable for bulk baking and freezing. You can also buy excellent poppadoms that you can heat up in the microwave. Most supermarkets stock them and they usually contain only a small trace of fat, though they can be a bit salty. Just heat them for a minute or so and your Indian meal is complete. For a proper home-made curry when you have more time, see pages 93–4.

Vegetable or meat lasagne

You can make either a vegetable lasagne, layering Ratatouille with no-cook lasagne pasta sheets, or a meat one with Ratatouille and Ragù meat sauce (pages 96–7 and 97), made and frozen earlier. See the Vegetable lasagne recipe (pages 98–9) for preparation instructions.

Cauliflower cheese
Serves 2

This recipe is made with low-fat (less than 16 per cent) strong mature cheese and provides an excellent quick meal for two or, if you double the quantities, for four. Although cheese tends to be high in fat, using the type of cheese selected for this recipe keeps the total fat level down to around 5 grams per portion. You can use a cheese that has more fat if you prefer, but remember to adjust the nutritional analysis if you need to check on fat levels.

Try making this recipe using half cauliflower and half broccoli. You'll still get the taste of the traditional recipe, but you'll give the meal a boost of vitamin C.

Ingredients
50 g (2 oz) quick-cook pasta
florets from $\frac{1}{2}$ good-sized
    cauliflower

For the sauce
1 heaped tbsp flour
1 level tsp mustard powder or
    paste
225 ml ($\frac{1}{2}$ pint) soya or semi-
    skimmed milk

40 g ($1\frac{1}{2}$ oz) low-fat mature
    cheese, grated
freshly ground black pepper
$\frac{1}{2}$ tsp paprika
1 tomato, sliced

Nutritional analysis
Per serving, 275 kcals (1155 kJ), 5 g fat, of which 2 g saturated, 210 mg sodium.

Method
1 Place the pasta in a saucepan of boiling water. Steam the cauliflower florets on top in a metal 'petal' steamer or cook separately. Put the lid on and cook for 10–12 minutes, then drain and set to one side.

2 While the cauliflower and pasta are cooking, make the sauce. Put the flour and mustard into a saucepan. Pour the milk in a little at a time and, over a medium heat and using a balloon whisk, mix until smooth. Turn up the heat and add the grated cheese, whisking all the time. Add black pepper to taste. As the mixture comes to the boil, it should turn into a thick pouring sauce. If it is too stiff, add a little more milk. If it is too runny, add a sprinkling of extra flour and whisk until it thickens.

3 Place the pasta in two serving bowls, add the cauliflower florets, then pour the sauce over the top.

4 Sprinkle a little paprika over and decorate with the slices of tomato. Serve with a portion of baked beans, tomato ketchup and a piece of toast, without spread.

Daal bhaat
Serves 2 or 4 with other dishes

The staple diet in Nepal, this light main dish is nutritious, easy to make and very tasty. This recipe is actually for the daal – bhaat refers to the rice with which it is served.

Lentils are an excellent source of cholesterol-lowering soluble fibre and, as a food with a low glycaemic index, they help to decrease the risk of diabetes and heart disease (see Chapter 2).

Ingredients

2 tsp olive oil
1 small onion, peeled and
  finely chopped
2 garlic cloves, crushed
1 tsp ground cumin
1 tsp ground coriander
2 tsp turmeric

1 fresh chilli, deseeded and
  finely chopped, or 1 tsp
  chilli powder
115 g (4 oz) red lentils
2 medium tomatoes, diced
570 ml (1 pint) water

To serve
rice, cooked
few sprigs fresh coriander, chopped

Nutritional analysis
Per serving, 114 kcals (479 kJ), 4 g fat, of which 1 g saturated, 20 mg sodium.

Method
1 Heat the oil in a large saucepan or flameproof casserole. Add the onion and garlic and fry gently for 5–6 minutes, until soft.
2 Add the cumin, coriander, turmeric and chilli. Cook for a further 2–3 minutes.
3 Rinse and drain the lentils, then stir them into the pan together with the tomatoes. Finally, add the water, bring to the boil and cook for about 20 minutes, or until the lentils have softened. Serve with the rice (bhaat) and fresh coriander.

Pancakes
Makes 6–8

Pancakes are a favourite worldwide. You'll find them in Chinese cookery and French – where they appear as crêpes or galettes – in addition to their crucial role in the traditional English pancake race. They're simple to make, very low in fat, if you follow this recipe, and provide an excellent basis for a whole range of creative snacks. Try them served simply with a squeeze of lemon juice and a sprinkling of sugar or be a bit more adventurous and fill them with apple, raisins and cinnamon or use a savoury filling, such as low-fat cream cheese and lightly cooked spinach or Ratatouille (pages 96–7).

Pancakes freeze well, but you'll need to place a sheet of greaseproof paper in between each one to make it easy to remove them individually later on.

Ingredients
115 g (4 oz) plain flour
1 egg
300 ml ($\frac{1}{2}$ pint) skimmed milk

splash light vegetable oil, for greasing

Nutritional analysis
For 6, per pancake, each 98 kcals (412 kJ), 2 g fat, of which 0.5 g saturated, 40 mg sodium.

For 8, per pancake, 74 kcals (311 kJ), 1 g fat, of which 0.3 g saturated, 30 mg sodium.

Method
1 Mix the flour, egg and milk together in a food processor or beat by hand until you have a smooth batter.
2 Spray or brush a frying pan with a little light vegetable oil. Set over a medium heat until the pan is nice and hot. Getting the pan hot enough first is one of the secrets of making good pancakes. You need very little oil, but you do need a hot pan.
3 Pour in enough of the pancake mix to coat the base of the pan thinly. You'll need to tip the pan from side to side to spread the mixture.
4 Cook for a couple of minutes or so, then flip or toss the pancake over to its other side. This is where the fun comes in! Cook for about 1 more minute, then turn out on to a warm plate.

Chocolate and pear pudding (from frozen)
Serves 2

In the Desserts section, on pages 116–17, is the recipe for these puddings. If you took our advice and made extra for freezing, you can feel rather pleased with yourself now because you need frozen ones for this.

Just place two puddings in the microwave and heat on high for 1 minute. Alternatively, you can reheat them in the oven. Simply place them on the middle shelf of an oven preheated to 170°C (325°F/gas mark 3), and bake for about 5–6 minutes.

The Chocolate sauce (pages 116–17) takes about 5 minutes to make from start to finish. Pour the sauce over the puddings and enjoy a magic moment!

Low-fat ice-cream with smoothie topping
Serves 6

Look out for one of the low-fat ice-creams that are available in the shops and place a small scoop of it in a wine glass as the base for your smoothie topping. The Strawberry smoothie (page 148) can be whipped up in a few minutes (omit honey for this recipe). The combination of ice-cream with the Strawberry smoothie makes a delightful special treat.

Nutritional analysis
Per serving, 116 kcals (487 kJ), 2 g fat of which 1 g saturated, 122 mg sodium.

Baked apple with mincemeat
Serves 1 apple per person

For a quick dessert, core a large cooking apple, prick the skin several times with a sharp knife or fork, fill the middle with 3 tsp Mincemeat (page 74) and microwave on full power for about $2\frac{1}{2}$–3 minutes per apple, so that the skin has softened a little. Then, place the apple or apples in an ovenproof dish or baking tray with a little water (2–3 tablespoons per apple) and bake in the middle of an oven preheated to 180°C (350°F/gas mark 4) for about 15 minutes.

The preparation time should be well under 20 minutes in total for a single apple and under 30 minutes for 4 – a lot less than the 45–50 minutes you would need to bake the apples in the oven from scratch. You can, of course, simply stick to using the microwave if you prefer. This is quicker, but you'll find that the skin will cook and taste a lot better if the apples are finished off in a conventional oven as described. Serve with custard, yogurt or low-fat ice-cream.

Nutritional analysis
Per baked apple with mincemeat, 345 kcals (1449 kJ), 6 g fat, of which 1 g saturated, 122 mg sodium.

Glossary

Alpha-linolenic acid *see* Omega-3 and omega-6 polyunsaturated fatty acids.

Angina Tight, cramp-like pain in the chest coming on with exertion or overexcitement, caused by a reduction in blood supply to the heart.

Antioxidants A collection of nutrients that are found in lots of fruits, vegetables and nuts, and also in wine, grape juice and tea. They help to prevent the oxidization of substances such as cholesterol. As cholesterol is much less likely to stick to the walls of our arteries in a non-oxidized state, antioxidants can help to stop our arteries from clogging up. They also help to prevent other diseases, including cancer, by mopping up *free radicals*.

Atherosclerosis Condition in which the arteries become furred up and narrowed, preventing the blood from circulating properly and leading to heart disease.

Cardiovascular system The heart and its related blood vessels.

Cholesterol A soft, waxy substance, mostly made in the liver from the fats we eat, especially saturated fat. It is a building block for all cell membranes, vitamin D and a variety of hormones, and is used to make bile, which helps in the digestion of food. There are two types of cholesterol – low-density lipoprotein (LDL) and high-density lipoprotein (HDL). If we have too much of the 'less desirable lipoprotein' LDL cholesterol, it can begin to clog up the arteries and lead to heart disease. The 'highly desirable lipoprotein' HDL variety, on the other hand, collects up surplus cholesterol and helps to keep the arteries clear.

Complex carbohydrates Starches, such as cereals, pulses, fruit and vegetables, and the main source of fibre in the diet. They are less readily available to our bodies for use as energy compared to simple carbohydrates, such as refined sugars and soft drinks, and are generally better for keeping our hearts in good shape.

Dietary cholesterol Cholesterol found in food – egg yolks, offal, shellfish and so on – but it is a relatively unimportant contributor to blood cholesterol levels compared to the cholesterol made by our bodies from the intake of fat, especially saturated fat.

Dietary fibre Fibrous food important for health. *Soluble* fibre, such as that in oats and beans, helps to lower cholesterol, while *insoluble* fibre, such as that in wholegrain bread and fruit and vegetables, helps to prevent bowel problems.

Familial hypercholesterolaemia (FH) An inherited genetic disorder in which levels of cholesterol are excessively high.

Fatty acids The constituents of fat. *See also* Omega-3 and omega-6 polyunsaturated fatty acids.

Flavonoids Potent antioxidants found in fruit and vegetables, wine, tea and chocolate.

Free radicals Chemical agents that encourage oxidization and are implicated in several diseases, including cancer. *See also* Antioxidants.

Glycaemic index (GI) A measure applied to foods indicating their effects on blood glucose levels. Foods with a *low* glycaemic index provide a slow and sustained release of glucose, increase levels of good HDL cholesterol and help to decrease the risk of diabetes and heart disease.

HDL cholesterol *see* Cholesterol.

Hydrogenation *see* Trans-fatty acids.

Hyperlipidaemia A condition in which blood lipid levels are raised.

Kilocalories (kcals) Measurement of calorie values, as found on food labels. The metric equivalents are *kilojoules (kJs)* and 1 kcal = 4.2 kJs.

Kilojoules (kJ) *see* Kilocalories.

LDL cholesterol *see* Cholesterol.

Linoleic acid *see* Omega-3 and omega-6 polyunsaturated fatty acids.

Linolenic acid *see* Omega-3 and omega-6 polyunsaturated fatty acids.

Lipids Collective term for a number of fatty substances in the body, including cholesterol.

Lipoproteins The tiny packages transporting cholesterol and other lipids to and from the body's cells via the bloodstream.

Mediterranean diet The type of diet typically eaten by people living in Mediterranean areas, including a range of fresh fruits and vegetables, the use of olive oil in cooking and the consumption of red wine. The diet is high in antioxidants and is generally considered to be beneficial to heart health.

Monounsaturated fats see Unsaturated fats.

Omega-3 and omega-6 polyunsaturated fatty acids *Omega-3* *fatty acids* are mainly derived from *alpha-linolenic acid* and are found, for example, in oily fish, vegetable oils such as rapeseed, and soya and their margarines, walnuts and leafy green vegetables. *Omega-6 fatty acids* are mainly derived from *linoleic acid* and found, for example, in sunflower, safflower, corn and soya bean oils and margarines. Keeping a good dietary balance between omega-6 and omega-3 fatty acids is important for heart health.

Plant stanols and plant sterols Ingredients extracted from plants that block the absorption of cholesterol into the body. They have been very successfully incorporated into margarines and other foods, such as yogurt and milk, and can be very effective in lowering cholesterol levels.

Polyunsaturated fats *see* Unsaturated fats.

Polyunsaturated fatty acids *see* Omega-3 and omega-6 polyunsaturated fatty acids.

Saturated fats Fats that are solid or semi-solid at room temperature. They are predominantly found in foods derived from animal origins, such as butter, lard, whole cream and fatty meats, and in 'hidden' fats in commercially baked products, such as biscuits, cakes, pies and confectionery. Too high an intake of saturated fats can lead to high levels of cholesterol, furred arteries and heart disease. *See also* Trans-fatty acids.

Trans-fatty acids Fats produced as a result of hydrogenation – the process used in converting unsaturated vegetable oils into solid fat for use in, for example, margarines and biscuits. Our bodies react to them as if they were saturates.

Triglycerides These are *lipids* and provide an important source of energy. Their volume is stimulated by intakes of fat and sugar and, if we have too many, they can lead to an increased risk of blood clots and coronary heart disease.

Unsaturated fats There are two types: *polyunsaturated* and *monounsaturated* fats. Unlike saturated fats, these help to *lower* cholesterol.

Useful books and websites

Books

Dr Robert Povey (2005) *How to Keep Your Cholesterol in Check*, 3rd edition, Sheldon Press.

This is the companion volume to *Eating for a Healthy Heart* and provides a comprehensive guide to the ways in which we can modify our cholesterol levels in order to achieve better heart health.

Paul Gayler with Jacqui Lynas (2003) *Healthy Eating for Your Heart*, Kyle Cathie.

Gourmet eating with heart-healthy ingredients.

Anthony Leeds, Jennie Brand Miller, Kaye Foster-Powell and Stephen Colagiuri (2003) *The New Glucose Revolution*, 3rd edition, Hodder Mobius.

A guide to the glycaemic index (GI) by nutrition experts at King's College, University of London, and the University of Sydney, Australia. Details of glycaemic index values given on the website at <www.glycemicindex.com> have also been compiled by these researchers.

Jacqui Lynas (2002) *Cooking for a Healthy Heart*, Hamlyn.

Isabel Moore (for the Food Foundation) (2002) *The Food Book: The essential facts about food and drink*, BBC.

A most informative guide to the origin and uses of a whole range of cooking ingredients.

Websites

H·E·A·R·T UK: www.heartuk.org.uk
British Dietetic Association: www.bda.uk.com
British Heart Foundation: www.bhf.org.uk
The Stroke Association: www.stroke.org.uk
Diabetes UK: www.diabetes.org.uk

Subject index

Recipe index

Further Titles from Sheldon Press

AVAILABLE NOW

How to Stick to a Diet
Deborah Steinberg and Dr Windy Dryden

Thousands of people go on diets, but the vast majority
give up without achieving their aims. The reason most
diets fail is because you lose sight of your long-term
goals. This book can help you get results from any diet,
using mental imagery, exercise and assertiveness to
change your behaviour and gain control of your eating.
It helps you identify and understand your personal
'danger points' where your will-power might weaken,
and strengthen your defences. Use this book alongside
any eating plan to add that vital extra ingredient for
success.

Price: 6.99   **ISBN: 0859697398**

Further Titles from Sheldon Press

AVAILABLE NOW

Living with Heart Disease
Victor Marks, Dr Monica Lewis &
Dr Gerald Lewis

Written by a patient, a doctor and a cardiologist, this
guide gives you the key information and advice you
need if:
- you have a family history of heart disease
- you have been diagnosed with a heart condition
- you suffer from angina

The good news is that heart disease is an illness that we
can control and in many cases actually reverse. This
doesn't come easily, but this book will help you
understand how your heart works and gives guidelines
for a lifestyle which will improve your health.

Price: 6.99   **ISBN: 0859698882**

Further Titles from Sheldon Press

AVAILABLE NOW

Living with Angina
Dr Tom Smith

Chest pain can be terrifying. Many people hope that if they ignore it, it will go away. But angina must be taken seriously, and it is very important to find out what you can about it. This book answers the key questions for anyone worried about angina: What should I do when I have chest pain? Does it mean I'm going to have a heart attack? How do I tell if it's serious? The book is also packed with useful advice about diet, exercise and lifestyle, to help anyone with angina live life to the full.

Price: £6.99   **ISBN: 0859697495**

Further Titles from Sheldon Press

AVAILABLE NOW

Living with High Blood Pressure
Dr Tom Smith

It's worrying to be told you have high blood pressure, especially if you have no symptoms and you don't feel ill. But it's important not to ignore the problem because of the risk of a heart attack or a stroke. This fully updated edition of *Living with High Blood Pressure* gives you the latest knowledge about the causes and effects of high blood pressure in a practical and reassuring way, and explains what you can do to help yourself. It also includes information about all the latest drug treatments, for handy reference about what your doctor prescribes, how it works and the possible side effects.

Price: 6.99   **ISBN: 0859698610**